Polyvagal Theory for Complete Beginners

A Quick-Start Guide to Understanding Your Nervous System and Finding Calm in Daily Life

Hanae Dakota Sparks

First Edition

ISBN (Paperback): 978-1-923604-32-2

ISBN (eBook): 978-1-923604-33-9

This book is for educational purposes only and is not intended as medical, psychological, or therapeutic advice. The information presented should not replace professional medical care or treatment. Always consult with qualified healthcare providers regarding any medical or psychological concerns.

The concepts presented are based on polyvagal theory as developed by Dr. Stephen Porges and related research. Some aspects of polyvagal theory remain subjects of ongoing scientific discussion and debate. References to researchers, clinicians, and their work (including Dr. Stephen Porges, Deb Dana, Dr. Bessel van der Kolk, and others mentioned) are for educational purposes only and do not imply endorsement of this work by these individuals.

The techniques and strategies described are intended for general wellness and educational purposes. Individual responses may vary, and what works for one person may not work for another. If you are experiencing persistent mental health difficulties, trauma responses, or other serious concerns, please seek appropriate professional support.

The author and publisher disclaim any liability for adverse effects arising from the use or application of the information contained in this book.

Table of Contents

Preface

You don't need another complicated book about your nervous system. You need practical tools that actually work, explained in ways that make sense, without the academic jargon or overwhelming complexity that makes most people give up before they start.

Polyvagal theory, which is one of the most useful frameworks for understanding how your body responds to stress and safety - has been trapped in dense textbooks and therapeutic settings for too long. The core insights are remarkably simple and immediately practical, but they've been buried under layers of technical language that make them inaccessible to the people who could benefit most.

Your nervous system is already working perfectly. It's doing exactly what it evolved to do - scanning for threats, mobilizing for action when needed, and seeking safety and connection when possible. The problem isn't that your system is broken; it's that modern life creates conditions your nervous system wasn't designed to handle. Understanding how it works gives you the ability to work with it rather than against it.

This isn't therapy, and it's not medical advice. It's practical education about how your body's automatic responses function and how you can support them more effectively. Some aspects of polyvagal theory remain subjects of scientific debate, which we'll acknowledge honestly. What matters is whether these concepts help you understand your own responses and develop tools that improve your daily experience.

You'll find no miracle cures here, no promises that breathing techniques will solve complex life problems, and no suggestion that nervous system awareness replaces professional help when you need it. Instead, you'll discover a framework that helps explain why you react the way you do in different situations and practical approaches that many people find genuinely helpful.

The information in these pages comes from decades of research by Dr. Stephen Porges and others, translated into everyday language and focused on immediate application. You can read this guide in less than thirty minutes and start using the concepts immediately. That's intentional - you don't need months of study to begin working more consciously with your nervous system.

Your nervous system has been taking care of you your entire life, often in ways you've never noticed or appreciated. Now you can learn to partner with it more skillfully. The tools are simple, the science is fascinating, and the applications are immediately relevant to whatever challenges you're facing.

Start wherever you are. Trust your own experience over any external authority, including this book. Use what helps, leave what doesn't, and approach your nervous system with the same respect and curiosity you'd bring to understanding any sophisticated system that supports your wellbeing.

Your nervous system is wise. Now you can become conscious partners in creating the kind of life you actually want to live.

Hanae Dakota Sparks

Chapter 1: Introduction - What Is This About?

Your Hidden Control System

Right now, as you read these words, something remarkable is happening inside your body. Without any conscious effort from you, an intricate biological system is monitoring your environment, adjusting your heart rate, managing your breathing, and making split-second decisions about whether you're safe or in danger. This invisible guardian never sleeps, never takes a break, and operates completely below the radar of your conscious awareness.

This system is called the **autonomic nervous system** (ANS), and it's arguably the most important biological process you've never really thought about.

Think of it this way: your ANS is like having a highly sophisticated security system installed in your body that's been running 24/7 since the day you were born. It's constantly scanning your internal state and external environment, asking questions like: "Is this person trustworthy?" "Is this place safe?" "Should I prepare to run or fight?" "Can I relax and connect with others right now?"

The fascinating part? This system makes all these determinations and triggers appropriate responses before your conscious mind even knows what's happening. You've probably experienced this yourself - walking into a room and immediately feeling uneasy without knowing why, or meeting someone new and instantly feeling comfortable in their presence. That's your autonomic nervous system at work.

Polyvagal Theory, developed by neuroscientist Dr. Stephen Porges over the past several decades, gives us a remarkably clear and practical way to understand how this system operates. Instead of viewing our nervous system responses as mysterious or unpredictable, polyvagal theory provides what amounts to a user manual for your own biological reactions.

But here's what makes this particularly interesting: once you understand how your autonomic nervous system works, you can actually learn to work with it rather than against it. You can begin to recognize your patterns, understand your triggers, and develop tools to help yourself feel safer, calmer, and more connected to others.

This isn't about suppressing your natural responses or trying to control everything your body does. Instead, it's about developing a partnership with your nervous system - learning its language, respecting its wisdom, and gently guiding it toward states that serve you better in your daily life.

The Key Insight: Biology First, Story Second

Here's the most important thing to understand about how your nervous system works, and it might surprise you: **your body decides how you feel before your mind creates a story about why you feel that way**.

Let me give you a concrete example. You're walking through a crowded shopping mall when suddenly you feel anxious. Your heart starts beating faster, your breathing becomes shallow, and you have an overwhelming urge to leave. What typically happens next? Your mind immediately starts searching for explanations: "There are too many people here," "The music is too loud," "I have too much to do today," or "I'm probably coming down with something."

But here's what actually happened: your autonomic nervous system detected something in your environment - maybe the lighting, the noise level, the density of people, or even someone's body language - and determined that this situation warranted a protective response. Your body shifted into a state of alert mobilization before your conscious mind had any idea what was happening. Then, because humans are meaning-making creatures, your brain quickly

4

constructed a logical explanation for the physical sensations you were experiencing.

This **biology-first, story-second** sequence happens constantly throughout your day, usually without you noticing it. You meet someone new and immediately feel wary - your nervous system detected something subtle in their facial expression or voice tone. You walk into your favorite coffee shop and feel your shoulders relax - your system recognized multiple cues of safety and familiarity. You check your email and feel your stomach tighten - your body responded to stress before you even read the message that's causing concern.

Understanding this sequence changes everything because it means you can start paying attention to what your body is telling you before your mind creates potentially inaccurate stories about what's happening. Your nervous system is incredibly sophisticated at detecting subtle environmental cues, but it's not always accurate in modern contexts. Sometimes it sounds alarm bells when you're perfectly safe, or fails to alert you when caution might be warranted.

The beautiful thing about polyvagal theory is that it gives you a framework for understanding these responses without judgment. Your nervous system isn't broken when it reacts to things that don't seem threatening to your logical mind. It's doing exactly what it evolved to do - keep you alive and help you navigate complex social environments.

What You'll Learn in This Guide

Over the next nine pages, you'll gain practical tools and insights that can transform how you understand and work with your nervous system responses. Here's what we'll cover together:

The Three Basic States Your Nervous System Can Be In

You'll learn about what polyvagal theory calls the "three-circuit system" - essentially three different biological states that your nervous system can activate depending on what's happening around you and inside you. These aren't complicated medical concepts; they're simple, recognizable patterns that you can learn to identify in real time. Think of them as different gears your body can shift into, each one designed for specific circumstances.

How to Recognize Which State You're In Right Now

Most people go through their entire lives without really understanding what their body is communicating to them. You'll learn to recognize the subtle (and not-so-subtle) signals that indicate which nervous system state you're currently experiencing. This awareness alone can be incredibly empowering because it gives you information about what's happening before your emotions become overwhelming or your thinking becomes clouded.

Simple, Research-Backed Ways to Shift Toward Feeling Safer and Calmer

This isn't about positive thinking or forcing yourself to relax. Instead, you'll learn specific, scientifically-supported techniques that work directly with your nervous system's natural tendencies. These include breathing practices, movement techniques, and ways of using your voice and environment to signal safety to your body. The best part? Most of these tools take just minutes to implement and can be used anywhere.

Why This Matters for Your Relationships, Work, and Daily Life

Understanding your nervous system isn't just personally beneficial - it can dramatically improve how you interact with others. When you know how to recognize and regulate your own states, you become better at helping others feel safe and calm too. You'll understand why certain people or situations consistently trigger you, and why others help you feel more like yourself. This knowledge can transform everything from how you handle workplace stress to how you connect with family members.

You'll also learn about something called "co-regulation" - the fascinating way that nervous systems influence each other. Once you understand this process, you'll see why being around calm people helps you feel calmer, and why your own regulated state can be a gift to others who might be struggling.

Important Note on Science

Before we go any further, I want to be completely transparent about something important: polyvagal theory provides an extremely helpful framework for understanding our nervous system responses, but like many theories in psychology and neuroscience, some of its specific claims are still being debated by researchers.

Dr. Stephen Porges, who developed this theory, has conducted extensive research over several decades, and many aspects of polyvagal theory are well-supported by scientific evidence. The existence and importance of the vagus nerve, the role of the autonomic nervous system in regulating our states, and the impact of breathing and social connection on our physiology are all firmly established in research literature.

However, some of the evolutionary claims about how these systems developed, and certain technical aspects of how the theory explains nervous system functioning, continue to be discussed and sometimes challenged by other neuroscientists. This is actually normal and healthy in science - theories evolve as we learn more, and ongoing debate helps refine our understanding.

What matters most for our purposes is this: regardless of which specific technical details might be refined or revised in the future, the practical applications of polyvagal theory have helped countless people better understand their responses and develop effective tools for regulation. Therapists, educators, healthcare providers, and individuals around the world have found this framework valuable for improving their well-being and relationships.

So as you read through this guide, focus on what feels useful and accurate to your own experience. If the three-state model helps you recognize patterns in your life and gives you tools for feeling more regulated and connected, then it's serving its purpose. Science will continue to evolve, but your personal experience of feeling more grounded and capable is what ultimately matters.

The goal isn't to become an expert in neuroscience - it's to develop a better relationship with your own nervous system so you can move through your life with greater awareness, compassion, and choice.

Chapter 2: The Three States - Your Internal Ladder

The Polyvagal Ladder

One of the most helpful ways to understand your nervous system is to imagine it as a ladder with three distinct rungs. This metaphor, popularized by clinician Deb Dana, makes it easy to visualize where you are at any given moment and how you might move between different states throughout your day.

Unlike a regular ladder where you climb up to accomplish a task, this nervous system ladder represents your body's automatic assessment of safety and threat. The fascinating thing is that you're always somewhere on this ladder - there's no "off" position for your autonomic nervous system.

Think of it this way: your nervous system is constantly asking, "How safe am I right now?" Based on the answer it arrives at (usually without your conscious input), it positions you on the appropriate rung of the ladder. Each rung comes with its own set of physical sensations, emotional tendencies, thoughts patterns, and behavioral impulses.

The three rungs, from top to bottom, represent progressively older evolutionary responses. The top rung is the newest system (in evolutionary terms), while the bottom rung represents our most ancient survival response. But here's what's important to understand: **none of these states are inherently good or bad**. Each one served our ancestors well in different circumstances, and each one still serves important functions in modern life.

Let's explore each rung in detail so you can begin to recognize these patterns in your own experience.

● VENTRAL VAGAL (Top Rung) - "Safe & Social"

How it feels: When you're in this state, the world feels manageable and you feel capable of handling whatever comes your way. You experience genuine curiosity about people and situations. Connection with others feels natural and appealing rather than draining or threatening. You might notice feeling calm but alert, creative, playful, or engaged. There's an underlying sense that "all is well" even when you're dealing with normal life challenges.

Your body: Your muscles feel relaxed but not limp - you have a sense of comfortable alertness. Your breathing flows easily and naturally without you having to think about it. Your heart rate is steady and calm. You might notice warmth in your chest or belly, and your face probably looks soft and approachable to others. Your voice tends to be melodic and expressive, and you make eye contact comfortably.

Your mind: Thinking feels clear and flexible. You can consider multiple perspectives on a situation without getting stuck in rigid thinking patterns. Problem-solving feels manageable rather than overwhelming. You're naturally curious about other people's thoughts and feelings. You can access humor and see the bigger picture even when dealing with difficulties. Learning new things feels engaging rather than threatening.

When it happens: This state often emerges when you're having dinner with people you care about and the conversation is flowing naturally. You might notice it when you're playing with children or pets, when you're absorbed in a hobby you love, or when you're learning something that genuinely interests you. It's the state you're in during good conversations, creative activities, or moments of genuine laughter. You might also experience it during gentle physical activities like walking in nature or practicing yoga.

Many people recognize this state from moments of deep connection - whether that's with other people, with nature, or with activities that feel meaningful to them. It's characterized by what researchers call "social engagement" - your face, voice, and body language naturally communicate safety and openness to others.

⬤ SYMPATHETIC (Middle Rung) - "Fight or Flight"

How it feels: This is your body's mobilization system, and it can show up in many different ways. You might feel energized and ready for action, anxious and keyed up, angry and ready to fight, or excited and stimulated. The common thread is activation - your system is preparing you to do something. This might feel like restlessness, urgency, irritability, or intense focus. You may feel like you need to move, act, fix, escape, or confront.

Your body: Your heart rate increases and you can probably feel it beating. Your breathing becomes faster and more shallow, or you might notice yourself holding your breath. Your muscles tense up, particularly in your shoulders, jaw, or stomach. You might feel hot or cold, and your hands could be clammy or shaky. Your voice may become faster, higher-pitched, or more intense. You might have trouble sitting still or find yourself fidgeting.

Your mind: Your thinking becomes laser-focused on problems, threats, or tasks that need immediate attention. You might find it difficult to see the bigger picture or consider multiple options - instead, your mind narrows its focus to whatever feels urgent. You may experience racing thoughts, worry loops, or an inability to concentrate on anything except what's bothering you. Creativity and humor often go offline, and you might find yourself thinking in black-and-white terms.

When it happens: This state activates when you're running late for an important meeting and can't find your keys. You'll recognize it during arguments or confrontations, when you're trying to meet a tight deadline, or when you're dealing with any situation that feels urgent or threatening. It also shows up during exercise (which is a healthy activation of this system), exciting events like concerts or sports games, or anytime you need extra energy and focus to handle a challenge.

The sympathetic state isn't automatically problematic - it's designed to give you energy and focus when you need it. The issue arises when you get stuck here chronically, or when this system activates in response to situations that don't actually require such intense mobilization.

⬤ DORSAL VAGAL (Bottom Rung) - "Shutdown"

How it feels: This state is characterized by a sense of disconnection, numbness, or emptiness. You might feel hopeless, defeated, or like nothing really matters. There's often a quality of "checking out" mentally or emotionally. You may feel invisible, unimportant, or like you're watching your life from a distance. Depression often involves spending significant time in this state, though you can visit it briefly during overwhelming situations without being clinically depressed.

Your body: Energy feels low or completely drained. Your body may feel heavy, like it's difficult to move or even lift your arms. You might feel cold, particularly in your hands and feet. Your breathing can become very shallow, and your voice may sound flat or monotone. You might slouch or collapse inward, and making eye contact with others feels difficult or impossible. Sometimes people describe feeling "foggy" or "underwater."

Your mind: Thinking often becomes slow and unclear. It's hard to make decisions, even simple ones like what to eat for lunch. You might experience what people describe as "brain fog" - difficulty concentrating, remembering things, or following conversations. Thoughts can become very self-critical or hopeless. You may find yourself thinking things like "What's the point?" or "Nothing I do matters." Problem-solving feels impossible, and the future can seem bleak or non-existent.

When it happens: This state often emerges after overwhelming experiences - receiving devastating news, dealing with prolonged stress, or facing situations that feel impossible to handle. You might notice it after intense arguments, during periods of grief, or when you're dealing with chronic illness or pain. Some people experience it during medical procedures, after accidents, or in response to feeling criticized or rejected. It can also show up when you're simply overwhelmed by too much stimulation or too many demands.

Unlike the sympathetic response which mobilizes you for action, the dorsal response is about conservation and protection through withdrawal. In extreme situations, this can be life-saving - but when it becomes a chronic pattern, it can significantly impact your quality of life and relationships.

Key Points About the Ladder

These aren't "good" or "bad" states - they're survival responses. Each rung of the ladder served important functions for our ancestors and continues to serve important functions today. The ventral vagal state helps us connect, learn, and thrive in community. The sympathetic state gives us energy to handle challenges, exercise, and respond to genuine threats. The dorsal state helps us conserve energy and survive overwhelming situations.

You naturally move between states throughout the day. It's completely normal to shift between different rungs of the ladder based on what's happening in your environment and your internal state. You might wake up in ventral vagal, shift into sympathetic when you're running late, return to ventral during a pleasant lunch with a friend, and briefly visit dorsal if you receive stressful news in the afternoon.

Each state served our ancestors well in different situations. The ventral state helped our ancestors cooperate, share resources, and raise children together. The sympathetic state helped them hunt, escape predators, and respond to immediate threats. The dorsal state helped them survive situations where fighting or fleeing wasn't possible - essentially "playing dead" until the danger passed.

The goal isn't to always be on top, but to have choice and flexibility. A healthy nervous system is one that can move fluidly between states as circumstances require, and can return to regulation (usually ventral vagal) when the situation no longer demands a protective response. Problems arise when we get stuck in one state, or when our system consistently over- or under-responds to current circumstances.

Understanding this ladder gives you a simple way to check in with yourself throughout the day. Instead of getting caught up in complicated emotional analysis, you can simply ask: "Which rung of the ladder am I on right now?" This awareness alone often creates space for choice about how you want to respond to whatever you're facing.

Chapter 3: Neuroception - Your Internal Smoke Detector

How Your Body Decides: Safe or Dangerous?

Right now, as you read these words, something extraordinary is happening beneath your conscious awareness. Your nervous system is conducting a sophisticated surveillance operation, continuously scanning your environment and your internal state for information about safety and threat. This process happens so automatically and so rapidly that you're usually completely unaware it's occurring.

Dr. Stephen Porges coined the term *neuroception* to describe this unconscious detection system that operates below the level of conscious awareness (Porges, 2004). Think of neuroception as your body's built-in smoke detector - except instead of just detecting smoke, it's constantly evaluating hundreds of subtle cues to determine whether your current situation is safe, dangerous, or somewhere in between.

Here's what makes neuroception so fascinating: it happens before conscious thought. Your body makes decisions about safety and threat before your thinking mind has any idea what's going on. You walk into a room and immediately feel uneasy, but you can't put your finger on why. You meet someone new and instantly feel comfortable with them, even though you've never spoken before. You're sitting in your own living room when suddenly you feel on edge, despite nothing obviously changing in your environment.

This isn't intuition or mystical thinking - it's your nervous system processing enormous amounts of information at lightning speed and arriving at conclusions about your safety before your conscious mind catches up.

But here's where it gets particularly interesting: your neuroception system can be influenced by your past experiences, your current physical state, and even your cultural background. This means that two people can be in exactly the same situation and have completely different neuroceptive responses. One person's nervous system might detect safety where another's detects danger, and both responses could be completely understandable given their unique histories and circumstances.

Understanding neuroception changes everything because it helps explain why you sometimes react to situations in ways that don't make logical sense to your thinking mind. Your body isn't malfunctioning when it sounds alarm bells in situations that seem perfectly safe to others. It's doing exactly what it's designed to do - keep you alive by erring on the side of caution.

What Your System Scans

Your neuroception system is constantly gathering and processing information from three main sources. Think of these as different channels of input that your nervous system monitors simultaneously, like a security system with multiple types of sensors.

Environmental Factors

Your nervous system pays close attention to the physical characteristics of your environment, often picking up on details that your conscious mind completely misses.

Lighting plays a surprisingly significant role in how safe you feel. Research has shown that bright, natural lighting generally promotes feelings of safety and alertness, while dim or harsh artificial lighting can trigger subtle stress responses (Berson et al., 2002). Your nervous system might react differently to the fluorescent lighting in an office building compared to the warm glow of candles at dinner, even if you're not consciously aware of the difference.

Sound and noise levels provide constant information to your neuroception system. Sudden loud noises typically trigger immediate

16

protective responses - that's why you might jump when someone drops a book, even when you know you're perfectly safe. But your system also responds to more subtle acoustic information: the gentle hum of conversation in a coffee shop might signal safety and social connection, while the jarring sounds of traffic or construction might keep your system slightly activated even when you're not consciously bothered by the noise.

Spatial characteristics of your environment matter enormously to your sense of safety. Your nervous system naturally prefers spaces where you can see exits, where you're not trapped or cornered, and where you have some control over who can approach you. This is why many people instinctively prefer to sit with their backs to a wall in restaurants, or why open office layouts can feel stressful even when they're designed to promote collaboration.

Familiar versus unfamiliar environments trigger very different neuroceptive responses. Your childhood bedroom probably feels safe in a way that a hotel room never quite does, even if the hotel room is objectively more comfortable and secure. Your nervous system has learned that familiar environments are typically safer than unfamiliar ones, so it relaxes more completely in spaces it knows.

People and Social Cues

Human beings are exquisitely tuned to detect safety and danger signals from other people. Your neuroception system is constantly reading micro-expressions, voice tones, body language, and other social cues to determine whether the people around you are safe to be with.

Facial expressions provide enormous amounts of information to your nervous system. Research has demonstrated that we can detect genuine versus fake smiles in milliseconds, often before we're consciously aware we're even looking at someone's face (Ekman, 2003). Your system responds differently to soft, relaxed facial features compared to tense, closed expressions. Even subtle changes around someone's eyes can signal to your nervous system whether that person feels safe and calm or stressed and potentially threatening.

Voice tone and prosody - the melody and rhythm of speech - communicate safety or danger information directly to your nervous system. A calm, melodic voice with natural variation in pitch tends to signal safety, while harsh, monotone, or high-pitched voices can trigger subtle defensive responses. This is why the way someone says "How are you?" can make you feel either welcomed or wary, regardless of the actual words they use.

Body language and posture provide continuous information about other people's internal states. Open postures with relaxed shoulders and uncrossed arms generally signal safety, while closed postures, crossed arms, or tense positioning can trigger protective responses in your nervous system. The distance people maintain from you, how they move through space, and whether their movements seem fluid or jerky all contribute to your neuroceptive assessment of their safety.

Eye contact patterns play a crucial role in social neuroception. Appropriate eye contact that feels genuine and non-threatening typically promotes feelings of safety and connection. But too much eye contact can feel aggressive or intrusive, while too little can signal disinterest or deception. Your nervous system has learned complex patterns about what constitutes "safe" eye contact based on your cultural background and personal experiences.

Internal Cues

Your neuroception system doesn't just monitor external threats - it also pays close attention to signals from inside your own body, using this information to determine how well-equipped you are to handle whatever challenges might arise.

Physical comfort levels significantly influence your sense of safety. When you're hungry, tired, too hot, too cold, or in physical pain, your nervous system interprets these states as potential vulnerabilities that make you less capable of responding to threats. This is why you might feel more emotionally reactive or socially sensitive when you're physically uncomfortable, even in situations that would normally feel completely manageable.

Energy levels and fatigue provide important information to your neuroception system about your current capacity to handle stress. When you're well-rested and energetic, your system allows for more social engagement and exploration. When you're exhausted, the same nervous system becomes more conservative, more likely to detect potential threats, and more inclined to seek safety and rest.

Memories and associations triggered by current circumstances can dramatically influence your neuroceptive response. A particular smell, sound, or visual cue that reminds your nervous system of a previous difficult experience can trigger protective responses even when your current situation is perfectly safe. This isn't your system malfunctioning - it's using past information to try to keep you safe in the present.

The remarkable thing about neuroception is how all these different streams of information get processed simultaneously and unconsciously, resulting in an overall assessment that gets translated into your position on the polyvagal ladder we discussed earlier.

Common Safety Cues

Learning to recognize what typically signals safety to your nervous system can help you understand your own responses and create environments that support your wellbeing. While individual responses vary based on personal history and cultural background, research has identified several universal safety cues that tend to promote ventral vagal activation across different populations.

Soft eye contact and genuine smiles represent perhaps the most powerful social safety cues available to humans. Research by Paul Ekman and others has shown that genuine smiles - those that involve both the mouth and the muscles around the eyes - trigger automatic responses in observers that promote feelings of safety and connection

(Ekman, 2003). Your nervous system has learned to recognize these expressions as indicators that the other person is in a calm, non-threatening state themselves.

Calm, melodic voices with natural variation in pitch and rhythm signal to your nervous system that the speaker is regulated and safe to be around. This is why listening to certain people speak can feel inherently soothing, while other voices might put you on edge even when the content of their words is perfectly benign. The prosodic features of speech - its musical qualities - communicate directly to your nervous system below the level of conscious awareness.

Open body postures with relaxed shoulders, uncrossed arms, and fluid movements typically signal safety and non-aggression. When someone approaches you with an open posture, moving slowly and predictably, your nervous system interprets these cues as indicating that this person doesn't pose a threat and might even be available for positive connection.

Familiar, comfortable environments where you know the layout, understand the social rules, and feel some degree of control naturally promote feelings of safety. This might be your own home, a favorite coffee shop you've been visiting for years, or any space where your nervous system has learned through repeated positive experiences that you can relax and let your guard down.

Feeling physically comfortable - being fed, rested, warm, and free from pain - provides a foundation of safety that allows your nervous system to engage with the external world. When your basic physical needs are met, your system has the resources available to connect with others and explore new possibilities.

Predictable routines and rhythms can also signal safety to your nervous system. Knowing what to expect reduces the amount of vigilance your system needs to maintain, freeing up energy for connection and creativity. This is why many people find comfort in morning routines, familiar meal patterns, or predictable work schedules.

Nature and natural environments often promote feelings of safety and regulation, possibly because human nervous systems evolved in natural settings over millions of years. Research has consistently shown that exposure to natural environments can reduce stress hormones and promote recovery from mental fatigue (Kaplan & Kaplan, 1989).

Common Danger Cues

Understanding what typically triggers protective responses can help you make sense of your own reactions and develop compassion for your nervous system's attempts to keep you safe. Again, individual responses vary significantly, but certain cues tend to activate sympathetic or dorsal responses across many people.

Harsh voices or sudden loud noises can immediately trigger sympathetic activation, even when you know logically that you're safe. Your nervous system evolved in environments where sudden loud sounds often indicated genuine threats, so it maintains this rapid response system even in modern contexts where most loud sounds are harmless.

Tense or closed-off body language signals to your nervous system that someone might be in a defensive or aggressive state themselves, which could potentially make them unpredictable or threatening. Crossed arms, clenched jaws, rigid postures, or jerky movements can all trigger subtle protective responses, even when the person displaying these behaviors has no intention of causing harm.

Unfamiliar environments with no clear escape route can activate your nervous system's threat detection systems. This response makes evolutionary sense - our ancestors survived partly by being cautious in new territories where they didn't know the dangers or escape routes. Modern examples might include crowded elevators, unfamiliar buildings with confusing layouts, or social situations where you don't understand the rules or expectations.

Being hungry, tired, or in pain doesn't just make you feel uncomfortable - it also signals to your nervous system that you're in a potentially vulnerable state with reduced capacity to respond to challenges. This internal state of vulnerability can make your neuroception system more sensitive to external threats, real or perceived.

Reminders of past difficult experiences can trigger protective responses even when your current situation is completely safe. This might be a particular song that was playing during a difficult time, a smell that reminds you of a hospital, or even someone's laugh that sounds similar to someone who hurt you in the past. Your nervous system uses this information from past experiences to try to protect you from similar situations in the future.

Unpredictable or chaotic environments can keep your nervous system in a state of heightened alertness. When you can't predict what might happen next, your system maintains a higher level of vigilance to be ready for whatever might occur.

Social rejection or criticism triggers powerful protective responses in most people, possibly because social exclusion represented a serious threat to survival for our ancestors. Even mild social disapproval can activate stress responses that seem disproportionate to the actual threat level in modern contexts.

Why This Matters

Understanding neuroception fundamentally changes how you can relate to your own emotional and physical responses. Instead of judging yourself for feeling anxious in situations that seem safe, or wondering why you can't just "think your way" out of certain reactions, you can begin to appreciate the sophisticated and usually helpful work your nervous system is doing on your behalf.

Your neuroception can be influenced by past experiences. This is particularly important to understand if you've experienced trauma, ongoing stress, or difficult relationships in your past. These

22

experiences can calibrate your neuroception system to be more sensitive to potential threats, leading to protective responses in situations that others might experience as perfectly safe. This isn't a character flaw or weakness - it's your nervous system doing exactly what it learned to do to keep you safe in previously challenging circumstances.

Someone with a history of trauma might detect danger signals where others see safety, while someone who grew up in a very secure environment might miss warning signs that others would notice immediately. Neither response is inherently right or wrong - they're both the result of nervous systems that adapted to their particular circumstances.

This creates opportunities for compassion rather than judgment. Understanding neuroception can help you respond to your own reactions with curiosity and kindness rather than criticism. Instead of thinking "I'm being ridiculous" when you feel uncomfortable in a situation that seems safe, you can ask "What might my nervous system be detecting that I'm not consciously aware of?"

This perspective also extends to other people. When someone seems to overreact to a situation or appears unnecessarily defensive, understanding neuroception can help you recognize that their nervous system might be responding to cues that you're not picking up on, or that trigger different responses in them than they would in you.

It provides a foundation for working with your responses rather than against them. Once you understand that your nervous system is constantly gathering information and making decisions about safety, you can begin to work in partnership with these responses rather than trying to override them through willpower alone.

This might involve learning to notice your neuroceptive responses more consciously, making environmental changes that support your sense of safety, or gradually exposing yourself to situations that challenge your nervous system in manageable ways.

23

Practice: Developing Neuroceptive Awareness

Throughout today, gently notice what makes you feel more or less safe. This isn't about changing anything or judging your responses - it's simply about developing awareness of how your nervous system responds to different cues.

You might notice that certain lighting makes you feel more relaxed, that particular people's voices affect your sense of calm, or that specific environments consistently influence your mood in predictable ways. You might observe that your responses change depending on whether you're hungry, tired, or well-rested.

The goal isn't to become hypervigilant about every sensation or overthink every response. Instead, you're simply developing a friendly curiosity about how your nervous system works, which can provide valuable information for supporting your own wellbeing and understanding your patterns of response.

This awareness often develops gradually over time. You might start by noticing obvious responses - like feeling immediately relaxed when you walk into your favorite coffee shop, or noticing tension when you're in a crowded, noisy environment. Over time, you may become more attuned to subtle shifts in your sense of safety and the environmental or social factors that influence these changes.

Understanding neuroception provides a foundation for all the practical tools and strategies we'll explore in the following pages. When you know how your nervous system gathers and processes information about safety and threat, you can begin to work with these natural processes to support your wellbeing and improve your relationships with others.

Chapter 4: Your Personal Nervous System Map

Recognizing Your Patterns

Your nervous system is as unique as your fingerprint. While we all share the same basic three-state structure, the specific ways these states show up in your body, thoughts, and behaviors are entirely your own. Learning to recognize your personal patterns is like getting to know a close friend - it takes time, attention, and gentle curiosity, but the insights you gain can transform how you move through your daily life.

Most people go through their entire lives without really understanding what their body is trying to communicate to them. They might notice that they feel "stressed" or "upset" or "fine," but they don't have a detailed map of how these states actually manifest in their specific experience. This is like trying to navigate a new city without a map - you might eventually get where you're going, but you'll probably take some unnecessary detours and miss opportunities along the way.

Creating your personal nervous system map involves paying attention to patterns across three key areas: what's happening in your body, what's happening in your mind, and what behaviors tend to emerge in each state. You'll also want to identify your unique triggers (what sends you down the ladder) and your glimmers (what brings you up the ladder).

This process isn't about becoming hypervigilant or constantly monitoring yourself. Instead, it's about developing a friendly awareness that can give you valuable information about what you need in any given moment. When you know your patterns, you can make choices about how to respond rather than feeling at the mercy of whatever state you happen to be in.

The worksheets that follow are designed to help you map your personal nervous system patterns. There are no right or wrong answers here - only your unique experience. Some people have very dramatic differences between states, while others notice more subtle shifts. Some people move quickly between states, while others tend to stay in one state for longer periods. All of these patterns are normal and valuable to understand.

VENTRAL VAGAL - When I Feel Safe & Connected

This is your state of safety and social connection, when your nervous system has determined that you're safe and that other people are available for positive interaction. Understanding how this state shows up for you personally can help you recognize when you're here and create conditions that support you in returning to this state when you've moved away from it.

My body feels: Pay attention to the physical sensations that characterize your ventral vagal state. This might include specific areas of relaxation or warmth, particular breathing patterns, or characteristic energy levels. Some people notice their shoulders dropping, their breathing becoming deeper and more natural, or a sense of warmth in their chest or belly. Others might notice that their muscles feel relaxed but alert, or that they have a sense of physical ease and comfort.

You might also notice what happens with your voice when you're in this state. Many people find that their voice becomes more melodic and expressive, with natural variation in tone and pitch. Your face might feel soft and relaxed, and you might find that making eye contact with others feels natural and comfortable.

My thoughts are: In ventral vagal, thinking typically becomes clearer and more flexible. You might notice that you can consider multiple perspectives on a situation without getting stuck in rigid thinking patterns. Problem-solving often feels manageable rather than overwhelming, and you might find yourself naturally curious about other people's thoughts and experiences.

26

Creative thinking often flows more easily in this state, and you might notice that you can access humor and see the bigger picture even when dealing with normal life challenges. Learning new things typically feels engaging rather than threatening when your nervous system is in this regulated state.

I tend to: The behaviors that emerge from ventral vagal tend to be oriented toward connection, creativity, and constructive action. You might notice that you're more likely to reach out to friends, engage in creative activities, or tackle projects that require focused attention. Play often feels appealing in this state, whether that's physical play, intellectual play, or social play.

You might also notice that you're more generous with others, more willing to be vulnerable or authentic, and more capable of setting healthy boundaries when needed. Conflict resolution often feels more manageable from this state because you can access empathy for other people's perspectives while still maintaining your own position.

This usually happens when: Understanding the conditions that typically support your ventral vagal state can help you create more opportunities to experience this regulation. This might include specific relationships that help you feel safe and understood, particular activities that engage you in positive ways, or certain environments that naturally promote feelings of safety and connection.

You might notice that this state emerges during certain times of day, or when particular physical needs are met (being well-rested, well-fed, or physically comfortable). Some people find that they access this state more easily in nature, while others find it in cozy indoor environments. Pay attention to both the external conditions and internal factors that tend to support your sense of safety and connection.

SYMPATHETIC - When I'm Activated

Your sympathetic state provides energy and focus for dealing with challenges, but it can also show up when your nervous system detects threat or stress. Understanding how sympathetic activation manifests for you can help you distinguish between helpful activation (like when you're exercising or excited about something) and protective activation (like when you're feeling threatened or overwhelmed).

My body feels: Sympathetic activation typically involves some form of mobilization - your body preparing for action. This might include increased heart rate that you can actually feel, changes in breathing (faster, shallower, or breath-holding), or muscle tension in particular areas like your shoulders, jaw, or stomach.

You might notice temperature changes - feeling hot or cold, having clammy hands, or experiencing fluctuations in your body temperature. Your voice might become faster, higher-pitched, or more intense than usual. Some people notice restlessness or an inability to sit still, while others might experience shakiness or trembling.

Energy levels in sympathetic can feel quite different depending on the context. Positive sympathetic activation (like excitement or healthy challenge) might feel energizing and invigorating, while protective sympathetic activation might feel draining or agitating.

My thoughts are: Sympathetic activation typically narrows your focus, which can be helpful when you need to concentrate on specific tasks or challenges. However, this narrowed focus can also mean that you lose sight of the bigger picture or have trouble considering multiple options.

You might notice racing thoughts, worry loops, or an inability to concentrate on anything except what's bothering you. Thinking often becomes more black-and-white, and you might find it difficult to access creativity or humor. Your mind might become laser-focused on problems, threats, or tasks that feel urgent.

In positive sympathetic activation, this focused thinking can help you accomplish tasks efficiently or perform well in challenging situations.

In protective sympathetic activation, the same mental patterns can feel overwhelming or unproductive.

I tend to: The behaviors that emerge from sympathetic activation are oriented toward action, although the specific actions can vary significantly depending on whether this is positive or protective activation. You might notice increased productivity, a tendency to move faster, or an urge to fix, escape, or confront whatever is triggering the activation.

Some people become more talkative in sympathetic states, while others might become more argumentative or irritable. You might notice a tendency to multitask, an inability to relax or rest, or an urge to keep moving or staying busy. In protective sympathetic states, you might notice controlling behaviors, conflict avoidance, or attempts to manage or fix other people's problems.

This usually happens when: Sympathetic activation can be triggered by both positive and challenging circumstances. Positive triggers might include exercise, exciting events, challenging but manageable tasks, or situations that require focused energy and attention.

Protective triggers might include time pressure, interpersonal conflict, overwhelming demands, or situations that remind your nervous system of previous stressful experiences. You might notice that this state emerges when you're dealing with deadlines, confrontations, or any situation that feels urgent or threatening.

Physical factors like caffeine, lack of sleep, hunger, or illness can also make sympathetic activation more likely or more intense. Understanding your specific triggers can help you prepare for situations that might activate this state and develop strategies for working with the activation rather than against it.

DORSAL VAGAL - When I Shut Down

Dorsal vagal activation represents your nervous system's conservation response when situations feel overwhelming or impossible to handle. This state can range from mild withdrawal to more complete shutdown, and it serves the important function of helping you survive situations that feel beyond your capacity to manage actively.

My body feels: Dorsal activation typically involves some form of withdrawal or decreased energy. You might notice your energy feeling very low or completely drained, as if moving your body requires enormous effort. Some people describe feeling heavy, like their limbs are weighted down, or feeling cold, particularly in their hands and feet.

Breathing often becomes very shallow in this state, and your voice might sound flat, quiet, or monotone. You might notice that making eye contact feels difficult or impossible, and your posture might naturally collapse inward or downward. Some people experience a sense of floating or disconnection from their body, as if they're watching themselves from a distance.

Digestion often slows down significantly in dorsal states, which might manifest as nausea, loss of appetite, or digestive discomfort. Sleep patterns might also be affected - either sleeping much more than usual or having difficulty sleeping at all.

My thoughts are: Thinking in dorsal states often becomes slow, foggy, or unclear. You might experience what people commonly call "brain fog" - difficulty concentrating, remembering things, or following conversations. Decision-making can feel impossible, even for simple choices like what to eat or what to wear.

Thoughts often become very self-critical or hopeless in this state. You might find yourself thinking things like "What's the point?" or "Nothing I do matters" or "I can't handle this." The future might seem non-existent or bleak, and it can be difficult to remember that you've felt differently in the past or that you might feel differently again.

Processing information becomes much more difficult in dorsal states. You might find that conversations feel overwhelming, that you can't follow the plot of a movie or book, or that simple tasks feel impossibly complicated.

I tend to: Behaviors in dorsal states are oriented toward withdrawal and conservation. You might notice a tendency to isolate yourself, avoid social contact, or withdraw from activities that usually feel engaging. You might spend more time sleeping, lying down, or simply staring into space.

Procrastination often increases in dorsal states, not because you're lazy or unmotivated, but because your nervous system is conserving energy for basic survival functions. You might find yourself "doom scrolling" on your phone, watching television for hours without really paying attention, or engaging in other passive activities that require minimal energy.

Communication often becomes minimal in this state. You might stop responding to texts or emails, avoid phone calls, or give very brief answers when people try to engage with you.

This usually happens when: Dorsal activation typically occurs after overwhelming experiences or when you're dealing with situations that feel impossible to handle through active responses. This might include receiving bad news, dealing with intense conflict, experiencing grief or loss, or simply being overwhelmed by too many demands at once.

Chronic stress, sleep deprivation, illness, or physical pain can all make dorsal activation more likely. Some people notice this state emerging after intense sympathetic activation - as if their nervous system needs to rest and recover after a period of high alert.

Certain environmental factors like overwhelming sensory input, social isolation, or feeling criticized or rejected can also trigger dorsal responses. Understanding your patterns can help you recognize when you might be vulnerable to this state and develop strategies for supporting yourself through it.

Your Triggers (What Sends You Down the Ladder)

Understanding what consistently moves you from more regulated states toward protective states gives you valuable information about

31

your nervous system's sensitivities. These triggers aren't character flaws or weaknesses - they're information about what your nervous system has learned to perceive as potentially threatening based on your unique history and experiences.

Situations: Think about specific types of situations that consistently trigger protective responses in your nervous system. This might include certain work scenarios like public speaking or performance reviews, social situations like large parties or family gatherings, or logistical challenges like running late or dealing with technology problems.

You might notice patterns around conflict, criticism, or feeling misunderstood. Some people find that unpredictable situations consistently trigger protective responses, while others are more affected by situations that remind them of previous difficult experiences.

Environmental factors like noise levels, lighting, crowding, or unfamiliar spaces might also be situational triggers for your nervous system. Understanding these patterns can help you prepare for challenging situations or make choices about which situations to engage with when you're feeling more or less resourced.

People/behaviors: Certain people or specific behaviors might consistently trigger protective responses in your nervous system. This doesn't necessarily mean these people are bad or harmful - sometimes it's simply a matter of nervous system compatibility or reminders of previous difficult relationships.

You might notice that you're triggered by people who speak loudly, interrupt frequently, or have closed body language. Some people are consistently triggered by criticism, even when it's constructive, while others might be more affected by people who seem unpredictable or emotionally intense.

Understanding these patterns can help you make conscious choices about relationships and develop strategies for interacting with people who trigger protective responses when you need to maintain those relationships for work or family reasons.

Physical states: Your physical condition significantly influences how likely you are to experience protective responses. Being hungry, tired, in pain, or ill can make your nervous system more sensitive to triggers that might not affect you when you're physically well-resourced.

Some people notice that certain foods, drinks, or substances consistently affect their nervous system regulation. Caffeine, alcohol, sugar fluctuations, or medication side effects might all influence your position on the polyvagal ladder.

Hormonal changes related to menstrual cycles, pregnancy, menopause, or other medical conditions can also influence your nervous system's sensitivity to triggers. Understanding these patterns can help you adjust your expectations and self-care strategies during times when you might be more vulnerable to protective responses.

Thoughts or memories: Certain thought patterns or memories might consistently trigger movement down the ladder. This might include thoughts about future challenges, memories of previous difficult experiences, or particular ways of thinking about yourself or your circumstances.

Some people notice that perfectionist thinking consistently triggers sympathetic activation, while thoughts about being a burden or worthless might trigger dorsal responses. Catastrophic thinking about potential future problems can also reliably activate protective states.

Understanding these cognitive triggers can help you recognize when your thinking patterns might be contributing to protective responses and develop strategies for working with these thoughts in more helpful ways.

Your Glimmers (What Brings You Up the Ladder)

Deb Dana coined the term "glimmers" to describe the opposite of triggers - the small moments, experiences, or cues that help move your nervous system toward safety and connection. Understanding your personal glimmers gives you a toolkit for supporting your own regulation and moving back toward ventral vagal when you've slipped into protective states.

Activities: Certain activities might consistently help you feel more regulated and connected. This might include physical activities like walking, dancing, or yoga, creative activities like drawing, writing, or playing music, or contemplative activities like meditation, prayer, or spending time in nature.

Some people find that organizing or cleaning helps them feel more regulated, while others find regulation through learning new things or engaging in challenging but manageable tasks. Social activities like having meaningful conversations, playing games, or sharing meals might also be reliable glimmers for your nervous system.

Understanding which activities consistently support your regulation can help you make conscious choices about how to spend your time and energy, particularly when you're feeling stressed or overwhelmed.

People: Certain relationships might consistently help you feel more like yourself and support your nervous system's sense of safety. These might be people who listen well, respond with empathy, or simply have a calming presence that helps you feel more regulated.

You might notice that some people help you access your sense of humor, creativity, or optimism more easily. Others might be particularly good at helping you feel understood or accepted just as you are. Understanding which relationships support your regulation can help you prioritize connection with these people during challenging times.

Places: Specific environments might consistently promote feelings of safety and connection in your nervous system. This might include natural settings like parks, beaches, or forests, or indoor spaces like libraries, coffee shops, or your own home.

You might notice that certain characteristics of spaces - like lighting, noise levels, or layout - consistently affect your sense of regulation. Some people find that organized, clean spaces support their nervous system, while others feel more regulated in cozy, lived-in environments.

Simple pleasures: Small, everyday experiences might reliably serve as glimmers for your nervous system. This might include sensory experiences like warm baths, soft textures, pleasant scents, or beautiful music. It might include simple rituals like morning coffee, evening tea, or lighting candles.

Food can also serve as a glimmer - not in the sense of emotional eating, but in the sense of nourishing yourself well and paying attention to which foods help you feel more grounded and energized. Understanding these simple pleasures can help you incorporate more regulation support into your daily routine.

Real Life is Complex

While the three-state model provides a helpful framework for understanding your nervous system, real life is often more nuanced than neat categories suggest. You might frequently experience what are called "mixed states" - combinations of different nervous system responses that occur simultaneously.

For example, you might feel excited about a new opportunity while also feeling anxious about the challenges it might bring (ventral + sympathetic). Or you might want to take action to solve a problem but feel too overwhelmed to move (sympathetic + dorsal). These mixed states are completely normal and provide important information about the complexity of your experience.

Some people also notice that they have different patterns depending on the context. Your nervous system might respond very differently at work compared to at home, or with family members compared to friends. You might have different triggers and glimmers in different seasons of the year or different phases of your life.

Understanding your patterns isn't about putting yourself in a box or limiting your experience - it's about developing awareness that can help you make more conscious choices about how you want to respond to different situations. Your patterns will likely continue to evolve as you grow and change, and that's exactly how it should be.

The goal is simply to develop a friendly relationship with your nervous system so you can work in partnership with it rather than feeling at its mercy. When you understand your patterns, you have more choice about how to care for yourself and how to move through your life with greater awareness and compassion.

Chapter 5: The Science - What Research Tells Us

Evidence-Based Understanding

Science is a process, not a destination. Our understanding of how the nervous system works continues to grow and change as researchers ask new questions, develop better tools, and challenge existing assumptions. This is particularly true in the field of neuroscience, where technological advances regularly reveal new information about how our brains and bodies actually function.

Polyvagal theory sits at an interesting intersection in this scientific process. Some aspects of the theory are well-supported by extensive research, while other components remain subjects of ongoing debate and investigation. This complexity doesn't diminish the practical value of the framework - it simply reflects the reality of how science works.

Dr. Stephen Porges first introduced polyvagal theory in the 1990s, and since then, hundreds of studies have investigated various aspects of the theory while thousands more have explored related concepts about nervous system functioning, stress responses, and the mind-body connection (Porges, 2011). What we've learned from this research provides both strong support for some key concepts and important questions about others.

Understanding what the research actually shows - and doesn't show - helps you make informed decisions about how to use this information in your own life. It also helps you maintain appropriate skepticism about any claims that go beyond what the evidence actually supports, while still appreciating the practical value of frameworks that help you understand your own experience.

The goal isn't to become a neuroscience expert, but rather to understand enough about the research base to use polyvagal concepts wisely and effectively. This means knowing which applications are well-supported by evidence and which ones are more speculative, so you can focus your energy on approaches that are most likely to be helpful.

What Research Strongly Supports

Several core concepts related to polyvagal theory have extensive research support from multiple independent research groups using different methodologies. These findings provide a solid foundation for understanding how your nervous system influences your thoughts, feelings, and behaviors.

The vagus nerve powerfully influences our sense of calm and connection. The vagus nerve is the longest cranial nerve in your body, connecting your brainstem to numerous organs including your heart, lungs, and digestive system (Breit et al., 2018). Research has consistently demonstrated that vagal activity is associated with feelings of calm, the ability to regulate emotions, and successful social engagement.

Studies using various measurement techniques have shown that higher vagal tone - generally indicating better vagal function - is associated with better emotional regulation, greater resilience to stress, and improved social functioning (Thayer & Lane, 2009). People with higher vagal tone tend to recover more quickly from stress, show better attention and cognitive flexibility, and report greater overall wellbeing.

Longer exhales than inhales activate the parasympathetic nervous system. This is one of the most consistently replicated findings in the research literature on breathing and nervous system regulation. When you extend your exhale longer than your inhale, you stimulate the parasympathetic branch of your autonomic nervous system, which promotes states of calm and recovery (Brown & Gerbarg, 2005).

Multiple studies have demonstrated that specific breathing patterns can measurably shift heart rate variability, blood pressure, stress hormone levels, and subjective reports of anxiety and well-being. This research provides strong support for using breathing techniques as practical tools for nervous system regulation.

Social connection and feeling safe measurably improve physical health. Extensive research has documented the profound impact of social relationships on physical health outcomes. People with strong social connections have lower rates of cardiovascular disease, stronger immune function, and longer lifespans compared to those who are socially isolated (Holt-Lunstad et al., 2010).

Research has also shown that feeling safe and supported can measurably reduce inflammation, improve immune function, and promote healing from both physical and psychological trauma. These findings support the polyvagal emphasis on safety and social connection as fundamental to wellbeing.

Early relationships shape how our nervous system develops. Decades of research in developmental psychology and neuroscience have demonstrated that early caregiving experiences significantly influence how children's nervous systems develop and function (Schore, 2001). Children who experience consistent, responsive caregiving tend to develop more flexible and resilient nervous system responses, while those who experience neglect, abuse, or inconsistent caregiving may develop nervous systems that are biased toward protection.

This research helps explain why people can have such different responses to similar situations - their nervous systems learned different lessons about safety and threat based on their early experiences. It also provides hope, because research shows that the nervous system remains capable of change throughout life in response to new experiences of safety and support.

Movement, breathing, and sound can shift our physiological state. Research across multiple fields has consistently demonstrated that specific physical practices can measurably influence nervous system functioning. Studies of yoga, tai chi, meditation, singing, and various forms of exercise have shown that these practices can reduce stress hormones, improve heart rate variability, and promote feelings of calm and wellbeing (Pascoe et al., 2017).

This research supports the practical application of embodied techniques for nervous system regulation and provides evidence for why approaches that work with the body - not just the mind - can be particularly effective for promoting wellbeing.

What's Still Debated

While many aspects of polyvagal theory align with well-established research findings, other components remain subjects of scientific debate. Understanding these areas of uncertainty helps you maintain appropriate perspective about what we know and don't know about nervous system functioning.

Some evolutionary claims about how these systems developed remain controversial among researchers. Polyvagal theory proposes a specific evolutionary sequence in which the nervous system developed, with newer systems layered on top of older ones. While this general principle of evolutionary layering is well-accepted, some researchers question the specific timeline and mechanisms that polyvagal theory proposes (Grossman, 2023).

These debates don't necessarily undermine the practical applications of polyvagal concepts, but they do suggest that some of the evolutionary explanations should be held lightly rather than accepted as established fact.

Whether specific measurements truly reflect "vagal tone" is an ongoing area of research and debate. Researchers use various methods to try to measure vagal activity, including heart rate variability, respiratory sinus arrhythmia, and other physiological markers. However, there's ongoing debate about which measurements most accurately reflect actual vagal functioning and what these measurements actually tell us about someone's nervous system state (Grossman & Taylor, 2007).

This technical debate doesn't affect the practical applications of polyvagal concepts, but it does mean that claims about measuring or improving "vagal tone" should be interpreted cautiously.

The precise mechanisms of how different vagal pathways work continues to be investigated and refined. Polyvagal theory proposes specific functions for different branches of the vagus nerve, but some researchers question whether these distinctions are as clear-cut as the theory suggests. Ongoing research is helping to clarify how different neural pathways actually function and interact.

Again, these technical debates don't necessarily impact the practical value of polyvagal concepts, but they do suggest that some of the mechanistic explanations may be simplified or incomplete.

Why This Matters

Understanding the current state of research on polyvagal theory helps you use these concepts more effectively and maintain appropriate perspective about their limitations and applications.

Science evolves, and honest scientists acknowledge limitations. Any theory in psychology or neuroscience should be understood as a work in progress rather than final truth. Polyvagal theory has contributed valuable insights and practical applications, but like all scientific theories, it continues to be refined and updated as new research emerges.

This doesn't make the theory worthless - it makes it human. Science progresses through proposing ideas, testing them, refining them, and sometimes replacing them with better explanations. The value of a theory isn't just whether every detail proves to be correct, but whether it generates useful insights and practical applications that help people.

Polyvagal theory provides a useful framework even while some details remain uncertain. Many frameworks in psychology and medicine are clinically useful even when we don't fully understand all the underlying mechanisms. Aspirin was used effectively for decades before scientists understood exactly how it worked. Similarly, polyvagal-informed approaches have helped many people better understand and regulate their nervous systems, regardless of whether every theoretical detail proves to be accurate.

Many therapeutic approaches based on this framework show positive results in clinical studies. Research has demonstrated the effectiveness of various interventions that incorporate polyvagal concepts, including trauma-informed therapy, breathing techniques, mindfulness practices, and somatic approaches (van der Kolk, 2014). These practical applications have solid evidence support, even if some theoretical aspects remain debated.

The Bottom Line

Focus on what helps you understand and work with your nervous system. If the three-state model helps you recognize patterns in your responses and gives you tools for feeling more regulated and connected, then it's serving a valuable purpose in your life. Science will continue to evolve, but your personal experience of greater wellbeing and more conscious choice in how you respond to challenges has value regardless of how theoretical debates ultimately resolve.

The most important question isn't whether polyvagal theory is perfect or complete, but whether it provides you with useful insights and practical tools for improving your life. Many people find that understanding the basic concepts - the three states, neuroception, the importance of safety and connection - helps them make sense of their own responses and develop more effective strategies for self-care and relationship building.

At the same time, maintaining some healthy skepticism about any theory or approach can help you avoid becoming overly attached to particular explanations or techniques. What matters most is finding approaches that actually help you feel more regulated, connected, and capable of responding to life's challenges with greater wisdom and choice.

Key Research Areas Supporting Core Concepts

Several broad areas of research provide strong support for the practical applications of polyvagal concepts, even when specific theoretical details remain under investigation.

Heart rate variability and health outcomes represent one of the most robust areas of research related to polyvagal concepts. Heart rate variability - the natural variation in the time between heartbeats - is considered an indicator of nervous system flexibility and resilience. Higher heart rate variability is associated with better emotional regulation, greater stress resilience, and improved overall health outcomes (Thayer et al., 2012).

Research has consistently shown that practices like meditation, yoga, slow breathing, and regular exercise can improve heart rate variability, while chronic stress, anxiety, and depression tend to reduce it. This research provides strong support for the practical application of nervous system regulation techniques.

Social connection and immune function research has demonstrated profound links between our relationships and our physical health. Studies have shown that people with strong social support have better immune function, lower inflammation levels, and reduced risk of numerous health problems (Cohen & Wills, 1985). Conversely, social isolation and loneliness have been shown to have health impacts comparable to smoking or obesity.

This research supports the polyvagal emphasis on social connection and co-regulation as fundamental to wellbeing, even if we don't fully understand all the mechanisms involved.

Breathing techniques for anxiety and depression have been extensively studied, with numerous randomized controlled trials demonstrating their effectiveness. Research has shown that specific breathing practices can reduce anxiety symptoms, improve mood, and enhance overall wellbeing (Zaccaro et al., 2018). These studies provide strong evidence for using breathing techniques as practical tools for nervous system regulation.

Trauma therapy incorporating nervous system awareness has shown promising results in numerous studies. Approaches that address both the psychological and physiological impacts of trauma - including EMDR, somatic experiencing, and trauma-informed yoga - have demonstrated effectiveness in helping people recover from traumatic experiences (Brom et al., 2017). This research supports the importance of working with the body, not just the mind, in healing and regulation.

Attachment research on co-regulation has provided extensive evidence for how humans influence each other's nervous system states. Studies of parent-child interactions, romantic relationships, and therapeutic relationships have demonstrated that calm, regulated individuals can help others become more regulated, while anxious or dysregulated individuals can trigger protective responses in others (Cozolino, 2014).

This research supports the practical importance of understanding co-regulation and developing skills for both regulating yourself and supporting others' regulation.

The research base supporting practical applications of polyvagal concepts continues to grow, providing increasing confidence in approaches that work with nervous system regulation to promote wellbeing. While theoretical debates continue among researchers, the practical value of these approaches for many people is well-documented and continues to be refined through ongoing research.

Understanding both the strengths and limitations of the current research helps you use polyvagal concepts most effectively - focusing on applications that have strong evidence support while maintaining appropriate perspective about areas that remain uncertain or speculative.

Chapter 6: Breathing - Your Most Accessible Tool

Evidence-Based Breathing Practices

Of all the tools available for working with your nervous system, your breath stands out as the most immediate, accessible, and powerful option you have. You can't always control your environment, you can't always change your circumstances, and you can't always influence other people's behavior - but you can almost always influence how you breathe.

This isn't just feel-good advice or ancient wisdom (though breathing practices have been used therapeutically for thousands of years). Modern research has provided compelling evidence that specific breathing patterns can measurably shift your physiological state, influence your emotional responses, and change how your nervous system interprets your current situation.

What makes breathing so effective for nervous system regulation is that it sits at the intersection of voluntary and involuntary control. Your breathing happens automatically without any conscious effort - your brainstem manages this process to keep you alive. But unlike other automatic functions like heart rate or digestion, you can also consciously influence your breathing patterns when you choose to.

This dual nature gives you a unique window into your autonomic nervous system. By changing how you breathe, you can send different signals to your nervous system about whether you're safe or threatened, calm or activated, present or distracted. Your body responds to these signals by adjusting other physiological processes accordingly.

The research on breathing and nervous system regulation is extensive and consistent. Studies have demonstrated that specific breathing patterns can reduce anxiety, improve mood, enhance focus, support immune function, and even influence gene expression related to stress and inflammation (Brown & Gerbarg, 2012). What's particularly exciting is that these changes often happen quite rapidly - you can experience shifts in your nervous system state within minutes or even seconds of changing your breathing pattern.

But here's what makes this really practical: you don't need special equipment, training, or ideal conditions to use your breath as a regulation tool. You can practice breathing techniques while sitting in traffic, before a difficult conversation, during a work break, or lying in bed. The simplicity and accessibility of breathing practices make them perfect tools for everyday nervous system support.

The Basic Science

Understanding how breathing influences your nervous system helps you use these techniques more effectively and gives you confidence in their power to create real physiological changes.

Longer exhales than inhales activate your "rest and digest" system. This is one of the most well-established findings in the research on breathing and nervous system function. When you extend your exhale longer than your inhale, you stimulate the parasympathetic branch of your autonomic nervous system - the branch responsible for recovery, healing, and restoration (Jerath et al., 2015).

Here's how it works: when you inhale, your heart rate naturally increases slightly. When you exhale, your heart rate decreases. This natural rhythm is called respiratory sinus arrhythmia, and it's actually a sign of a healthy, flexible nervous system. By extending your exhales, you enhance this natural process and tip your nervous system toward the parasympathetic state.

This isn't just theoretical - researchers can measure these changes using heart rate monitors, blood pressure cuffs, and other physiological indicators. People practicing extended exhale breathing show measurable decreases in stress hormones, blood pressure, and muscle tension within minutes of starting the practice.

Breathing through your nose engages different neural pathways than mouth breathing. Your nose isn't just a backup system for when your mouth is busy - it's actually a sophisticated biological filter and nervous system interface. Nasal breathing activates the parasympathetic nervous system more effectively than mouth breathing, partly because the air takes a longer, more complex path to your lungs, allowing for better oxygenation and CO_2 regulation (Nestor, 2020).

Nasal breathing also stimulates the production of nitric oxide, a molecule that has numerous beneficial effects including improved circulation, enhanced immune function, and better nervous system regulation. When you breathe through your mouth, you miss these benefits and may actually activate your sympathetic nervous system more than necessary.

Slow breathing (4-6 breaths per minute) promotes heart rate variability, a marker of resilience. Normal resting breathing typically happens at 12-20 breaths per minute, but research has shown that slowing your breathing to 4-6 breaths per minute creates optimal conditions for nervous system regulation (Zaccaro et al., 2018).

This slower breathing rate enhances heart rate variability - the natural variation in time between heartbeats. Higher heart rate variability is associated with better stress resilience, improved emotional regulation, and overall better health outcomes. When you breathe at this slower rate, you're essentially training your nervous system to be more flexible and responsive.

The beautiful thing about these breathing effects is that they're not dependent on belief, positive thinking, or perfect technique. They're biological responses that happen automatically when you change your breathing patterns. This makes breathing practices remarkably reliable tools for nervous system regulation.

Ventral Vagal Breathing - For Connection & Calm

When you want to move toward or maintain a state of calm connection - what we call ventral vagal activation - specific breathing patterns can help signal safety to your nervous system and promote the physiological changes associated with this regulated state.

4-7-8 Technique

This practice was popularized by Dr. Andrew Weil and has been studied extensively for its calming effects. The pattern creates a strong emphasis on the exhale, which powerfully activates your parasympathetic nervous system.

How to practice:

1. **Inhale through nose for 4 counts.** Place your tongue gently against the roof of your mouth behind your front teeth. Breathe in quietly through your nose while counting to four. Don't worry about making the counts perfectly timed - just use a comfortable, steady rhythm.

2. **Hold for 7 counts.** Gently hold your breath for a count of seven. If this feels uncomfortable, you can reduce the hold time or skip it entirely. The hold creates a brief period of increased CO_2, which can enhance the relaxation response when you exhale.

3. **Exhale through mouth for 8 counts.** Part your lips slightly and exhale completely through your mouth, making a gentle whooshing sound if it feels natural. This extended exhale is the most important part of the technique.

4. **Repeat 3-4 times.** This practice is quite powerful, so start with just a few rounds. With regular practice, you can gradually increase to 8-10 rounds if desired.

The 4-7-8 pattern is particularly effective before sleep, during anxiety episodes, or anytime you need to shift quickly from activation into calm. Many people find that practicing this technique regularly helps them fall asleep more easily and feel more relaxed throughout the day.

Box Breathing

Also known as square breathing, this technique creates a balanced, rhythmic pattern that promotes stability and calm focus. It's used by military personnel, athletes, and emergency responders to maintain calm under pressure.

How to practice:

1. **Inhale for 4, hold for 4.** Breathe in slowly through your nose for a count of four. Then hold your breath comfortably for another count of four.

2. **Exhale for 4, hold for 4.** Exhale slowly through your nose or mouth for a count of four, then hold empty for a count of four before beginning the next cycle.

3. **Continue for 2-5 minutes.** Start with shorter periods and gradually build up. You can adjust the count (3-3-3-3 or 5-5-5-5) based on your lung capacity and comfort level.

Box breathing creates a meditative rhythm that can help quiet mental chatter while promoting physiological calm. It's excellent for preparation before challenging situations, during work breaks, or as part of a daily mindfulness practice.

The equal timing of all four phases creates a sense of balance and control that many people find particularly soothing. If holding your breath feels uncomfortable, you can practice a modified version with just the inhale and exhale phases (4 in, 4 out).

Sympathetic Breathing - For Energy & Focus

Sometimes you need healthy activation rather than relaxation. Maybe you're feeling sluggish and need energy for a workout, or you're about to give a presentation and want alert focus without anxiety. Specific breathing patterns can help you access sympathetic activation in a controlled, intentional way.

Energizing Breath

This technique provides gentle activation that can help you feel more alert and focused without triggering anxiety or overwhelm.

How to practice:

1. **Equal inhales and exhales (4 in, 4 out).** Unlike the calming techniques that emphasize longer exhales, this pattern uses equal timing for inhale and exhale. This balance provides energy without overstimulation.

2. **Slightly faster pace.** Practice at a slightly quicker rhythm than you would for relaxation breathing, but not so fast that it feels forced or creates tension.

3. **Use when you need alertness without anxiety.** This is perfect for morning energy, pre-workout activation, or before tasks that require focused attention.

The equal inhale-exhale pattern prevents the strong parasympathetic activation that comes with extended exhales, while the slightly faster pace provides gentle sympathetic stimulation. This creates what researchers call "calm alertness" - being energized but not stressed.

You can practice this while walking, before exercise, or anytime you need a natural energy boost without caffeine or other stimulants. Many people find it helpful in the afternoon when they need to maintain energy but don't want to interfere with evening relaxation.

Moving From Dorsal - Gentle Awakening

When you're in a dorsal vagal state - feeling shut down, disconnected, or numb - forcing energetic breathing practices can sometimes feel overwhelming or even trigger more shutdown. Instead, very gentle approaches that honor your nervous system's need for safety often work better.

Simple Presence Breathing

This isn't really a technique so much as a gentle way of reconnecting with your breath and your body when you're feeling disconnected.

How to practice:

1. **Just notice your natural breath.** Without trying to change anything, simply become aware that you're breathing. You might notice the sensation of air moving in and out of your nose, the rise and fall of your chest or belly, or the natural pauses between breaths.

2. **No counting or changing.** Resist the urge to control or improve your breathing. The goal is simply gentle awareness and reconnection with this basic life process.

3. **If you can, make exhales slightly longer.** Only if it feels easy and natural, you might allow your exhales to become slightly longer than your inhales. But if this feels like effort, just stay with simple observation.

4. **Stop if you feel worse.** If focusing on your breath increases anxiety, disconnection, or any other uncomfortable sensations, simply return your attention to something else. Sometimes when we're in dorsal states, even gentle practices can feel overwhelming.

The key with dorsal breathing practices is titration - using the smallest possible intervention that might be helpful. For some people, this might mean just placing a hand on their chest and feeling the gentle movement of breathing. For others, it might mean breathing along with a loved one or pet whose breathing they can observe.

The goal isn't to force a state change but to create the gentlest possible reconnection with your body and breath. Often, this gentle approach naturally supports movement toward more regulation over time.

When to Practice

Breathing practices are most effective when you use them consistently rather than only during crisis moments. Think of them as tools for both prevention and intervention - practices that can help you maintain regulation and also help you recover regulation when you've lost it.

Before challenging conversations. Taking even one minute to practice calming breathing before a difficult discussion can help ensure that you stay in ventral vagal during the conversation. This makes you more likely to listen well, respond thoughtfully, and work toward productive solutions rather than getting caught in defensive reactions.

When you notice moving down the ladder. As you develop awareness of your nervous system patterns, you'll start noticing when you're beginning to shift into sympathetic activation or dorsal shutdown. This is the perfect time to use breathing practices to support yourself in returning to regulation before the state becomes entrenched.

As a daily practice (even 2 minutes helps). Regular breathing practice when you're already regulated helps strengthen your nervous system's capacity for regulation and makes it easier to return to calm states when you do get activated. Many people find that practicing for just a few minutes each morning sets a foundation for better regulation throughout the day.

When you wake up or before sleep. Your breathing naturally changes during sleep transitions, and conscious breathing practices can support these natural shifts. Morning breathing can help you start the day in a regulated state, while evening breathing can help signal to your nervous system that it's safe to rest and restore.

You might also use breathing practices during transitions throughout your day - before starting work, after coming home, before meals, or during breaks. These mini-practices can help prevent the accumulation of stress and maintain better overall regulation.

The most important thing is finding times and patterns that work for your life. Some people prefer longer practices a few times per week, while others like very brief practices multiple times per day. Experiment to find what feels sustainable and helpful for your particular circumstances and preferences.

Chapter 7: Movement & Sound - Embodied Regulation

Moving Your Way to Regulation

Your nervous system doesn't exist in isolation from your body - it IS your body's primary organizing system. This means that how you move, hold yourself, and use your physical form directly influences your nervous system state. Movement isn't just something your nervous system controls; it's also something your nervous system responds to and learns from.

This might seem backwards if you're used to thinking of emotions and thoughts as purely mental phenomena. But research in embodied cognition has shown that your physical posture, movement patterns, and even facial expressions can influence your emotional state and nervous system activation (Cuddy et al., 2015). Your body and nervous system are in constant conversation, each influencing the other in dynamic ways.

Different types of movement serve different nervous system states and can help you either maintain your current state or transition to a different one. Just as you can use breathing to shift your nervous system state, you can use specific movement patterns to support regulation, discharge excess energy, or gently awaken from shutdown states.

What's particularly valuable about movement practices is that they work with your nervous system's natural tendencies rather than against them. When you're activated, your body naturally wants to move - movement practices give you productive ways to honor that impulse. When you're shut down, your body needs gentle awakening - movement practices can provide that without overwhelming your system.

The key is matching the movement to your current state and your desired direction of change. Forcing yourself to do energetic movement when you're in dorsal shutdown rarely works well, just as trying to do restorative movement when you're highly activated might increase frustration rather than promoting calm.

Ventral Vagal Movement - Gentle & Connecting

When you're in ventral vagal or want to support movement toward this regulated state, certain types of movement can enhance feelings of safety, connection, and calm alertness. These movements typically share characteristics of being rhythmic, flowing, and pleasurable rather than goal-oriented or performance-focused.

Slow, flowing movements (gentle yoga, tai chi) work particularly well for supporting ventral vagal states because they combine gentle physical activity with mindful attention and natural breathing. These practices often involve movements that naturally massage your internal organs, stimulate your vagus nerve, and promote the kind of calm alertness that characterizes ventral vagal activation.

The flowing nature of these movements can help your nervous system settle into rhythms that promote regulation. Unlike vigorous exercise that's designed to challenge your system, gentle flowing movements work with your body's natural patterns and preferences.

Rocking or swaying taps into some of the most fundamental movement patterns for nervous system regulation. Think about how babies are naturally soothed by rocking, or how many adults instinctively sway when listening to music they love. These rhythmic movements seem to activate deep patterns in your nervous system that promote calm and connection.

You can rock in a chair, sway while standing, or even do gentle rocking movements while lying down. The key is finding a rhythm that feels naturally soothing rather than forced or mechanical.

Walking in nature combines gentle physical movement with the nervous system benefits of natural environments. Research has consistently shown that spending time in nature can reduce stress hormones and promote feelings of calm and well-being (Li, 2010). When you combine this with the gentle, rhythmic movement of walking, you create ideal conditions for ventral vagal activation.

The pace doesn't need to be fast or challenging - a gentle, comfortable walking speed often works better for nervous system regulation than more vigorous hiking or power walking.

Dancing to music you love can be incredibly effective for promoting ventral vagal states, especially when you focus on pleasure and expression rather than performance or technique. Dancing engages multiple systems simultaneously - movement, rhythm, music, and often social connection if you're dancing with others.

The key is choosing music and movements that feel good to your body rather than pushing yourself to dance in particular ways. Let your body move in whatever way feels natural and enjoyable.

Playing with pets or children naturally promotes ventral vagal activation because it combines movement with social connection and often includes elements of play and humor. These interactions typically involve the kind of spontaneous, unstructured movement that your nervous system finds regulating.

The shared joy and connection that often arise during play can enhance the nervous system benefits of the physical movement itself.

Sympathetic Movement - Discharging Energy

When you're in sympathetic activation, your nervous system has mobilized energy for action. Sometimes the most effective way to work with this activation is to give your body appropriate outlets for this energy rather than trying to force yourself into calm states.

Vigorous exercise (running, jumping, sports) can be excellent for working with sympathetic activation, especially when the activation is related to stress or anxiety rather than genuine threats. Your nervous system has prepared your body for physical action, and providing that action can help complete the stress cycle and allow your system to return to regulation.

The key is using exercise as a tool for nervous system regulation rather than as punishment or a way to exhaust yourself. The goal is to move the energy through your system in a way that feels good and helps you return to calm rather than creating additional stress.

Shaking or trembling (let your body vibrate naturally) is one of the most natural ways to discharge nervous system activation. Many animals shake after escaping from predators, and humans have this same capacity for releasing stored stress and tension through spontaneous movement.

You can encourage natural shaking by simply standing and allowing your body to vibrate or tremble in whatever way feels natural. This might start small - perhaps just shaking your hands or shoulders - and can expand to involve your whole body if that feels good.

Push-ups against a wall or other forms of resistance movement can provide an outlet for sympathetic energy while giving you a sense of strength and capability. The resistance provides your muscles with something to push against, which can be satisfying when your nervous system is activated.

Dancing to upbeat music can help you move sympathetic energy in joyful, expressive ways. Unlike the gentle dancing that supports ventral vagal states, this might involve more energetic, vigorous movements that help discharge activation while still being enjoyable and self-expressive.

Any movement that feels like "getting energy out" can be effective. This might include jumping jacks, running up and down stairs, vigorous cleaning, or any other movement that helps you feel like you're productively using the energy your nervous system has mobilized.

The important thing is that the movement feels satisfying and helps you feel more settled afterward rather than more agitated.

Dorsal Movement - Gentle Awakening

When you're in dorsal vagal shutdown, your nervous system has essentially gone offline to protect you from overwhelm. Movement practices for this state need to be extremely gentle and non-demanding, designed to gradually and safely reconnect you with your body without overwhelming your system.

Gentle stretching while lying down can provide a way to begin moving without requiring much energy or creating demands on your system. This might involve slowly stretching your arms overhead, gently pulling your knees toward your chest, or any other movements that feel easy and comfortable.

The lying-down position reduces the demands on your nervous system while still allowing for gentle movement and body awareness.

Slow walking can help gradually mobilize your system without overwhelming it. This isn't about getting exercise or going anywhere in particular - it's about gently engaging your body's capacity for movement and helping energy begin to flow again.

You might walk very slowly around your house, in your yard, or just back and forth in a hallway. The pace should feel sustainable and not effortful.

Simple arm movements like gently lifting your arms, making slow circles, or any other movements that feel easy and natural can help begin the process of reconnecting with your body. These movements can often be done while sitting or lying down, making them accessible even when you feel very low energy.

Touching your own arms or hands gently provides a combination of movement and self-soothing touch that can help begin to awaken your system. This might involve gently stroking your own arms, holding your own hands, or any other self-touch that feels comforting and connecting.

The key with all dorsal movement practices is to go very slowly and pay attention to your body's responses. If any movement increases disconnection or overwhelm, it's important to stop and perhaps try something even gentler or simply rest.

Sound & Voice - Your Internal Tuning Fork

Your voice and the sounds you make or listen to have direct connections to your nervous system through your vagus nerve and other neural pathways. This makes sound a particularly powerful tool for nervous system regulation, one that you can use almost anywhere and anytime.

Research has shown that specific sounds and vocal practices can stimulate the vagus nerve, influence heart rate variability, and promote different nervous system states (Kang et al., 2018). This isn't just about the psychological effects of music you enjoy - though those are real too - but about the direct physiological impacts of sound vibrations on your nervous system.

Calming Sounds

Humming or "OM" (stimulates vagus nerve) creates vibrations that directly stimulate your vagus nerve and can promote feelings of calm and connection. The vibration created by humming literally massages your vagus nerve from the inside, which is why humming often feels naturally soothing.

You don't need to hum any particular tune or make it sound good - just creating the vibration is beneficial. Many people find that humming while they do other activities like cooking or cleaning helps them stay more regulated throughout the day.

Singing softly can provide similar benefits to humming while also engaging your breath in supportive ways. Singing naturally encourages longer exhales, which activate your parasympathetic nervous system, and the vocal vibrations stimulate your vagus nerve.

Again, this isn't about performance or sounding good - it's about using your voice as a tool for nervous system support. You might sing along to songs you know, hum melodies, or even just make up sounds that feel good.

Classical music at 60-80 beats per minute has been specifically studied for its calming effects on the nervous system. This tempo roughly matches a calm resting heart rate, which can help encourage your own nervous system to settle into similar rhythms (Chanda & Levitin, 2013).

Nature sounds (ocean, rain, birds) often promote feelings of calm and safety, possibly because human nervous systems evolved in natural environments. These sounds can provide a calming background that supports regulation without being distracting.

Activating Sounds

Upbeat music matching your target energy can help you access healthy sympathetic activation when you need energy or motivation. The key is choosing music that promotes the kind of energy you want - focused and alert rather than anxious or agitated.

Clapping or drumming can provide rhythmic stimulation that helps mobilize energy in structured ways. The repetitive rhythmic nature of these sounds can help organize your nervous system while providing gentle activation.

Energetic singing can help you access and express activation in healthy ways. Unlike soft singing that promotes calm, more vigorous singing can help you work with sympathetic energy while still engaging your breath and voice in supportive ways.

For Shutdown

Very gentle music or silence often works best when you're in dorsal states. Loud or complex sounds can feel overwhelming when your nervous system is already shutting down, so simple, quiet sounds or even complete silence might be most supportive.

Soft humming can provide gentle vagus nerve stimulation without being demanding or overwhelming. The vibration can help begin to awaken your system gradually and safely.

Listening to a calm, caring voice - whether that's a friend, family member, guided meditation, or audiobook - can provide gentle stimulation and connection without requiring any effort from you. The human voice has particular power to promote feelings of safety and connection.

Practice Tips

Notice which movements feel good in different states. Your body's wisdom about what it needs is usually more accurate than any external prescription. Pay attention to what movements and sounds naturally appeal to you when you're in different nervous system states.

Trust your body's wisdom over rigid rules. While the guidelines above can be helpful starting points, your individual nervous system might respond differently. Some people find vigorous movement calming, while others find gentle movement energizing. Trust your own experience over any external authority.

Start small - even 30 seconds of movement can help. You don't need long, elaborate movement practices to influence your nervous system. Brief moments of movement throughout your day can provide significant support for regulation.

Use sound as background support for movement. Combining movement and sound practices can enhance the benefits of both. You might hum while walking, listen to music while stretching, or practice breathing techniques while listening to nature sounds.

The most important thing is developing a experimental, curious relationship with movement and sound as nervous system tools. What works for you might be different from what works for others, and what works for you might change over time or in different circumstances. The goal is building a personalized toolkit of practices that feel supportive and accessible in your daily life.

Chapter 8: Connection & Co-Regulation

The Biology of Relationships

Humans didn't survive and thrive as a species because we were the fastest, strongest, or most individually capable creatures on the planet. We made it because we figured out how to work together, support each other, and literally share our nervous system resources to help everyone in the group stay regulated and safe.

This isn't just a nice philosophical idea about the importance of community - it's a biological reality that's wired into your nervous system at the most fundamental level. Your autonomic nervous system doesn't operate in isolation from other people. It's constantly reading, responding to, and influencing the nervous systems of people around you through processes that happen completely below the level of conscious awareness.

Think about how you feel when you're around someone who's genuinely calm and present compared to how you feel around someone who's anxious and rushed. Or notice what happens to your own internal state when you spend time with a friend who helps you feel more like yourself versus time with someone who consistently leaves you feeling drained or on edge. These aren't just personality preferences - they're your nervous system responding to the nervous system states of others.

This process, called *co-regulation*, represents one of the most important but underappreciated aspects of human relationships (Schore, 2003). Understanding how co-regulation works can transform how you think about your relationships, how you show up for others, and how you choose to spend your time and energy.

Most people think of emotions and nervous system states as purely individual experiences - something that happens inside you in response to your thoughts, circumstances, or personal history. But research has shown that nervous system regulation is actually a fundamentally social process. You literally borrow regulation from others and offer regulation to them through mechanisms that operate automatically and unconsciously.

This means that your nervous system state affects everyone around you, and everyone around you affects your nervous system state. You're not separate from the people in your environment - you're part of an interconnected web of nervous systems that influence each other constantly.

Co-Regulation: How It Works

The science behind co-regulation involves several different biological mechanisms working together to create what researchers call "physiological synchrony" between people who are interacting with each other.

Your calm nervous system can help calm others. When your nervous system is regulated - when you're in ventral vagal - you naturally emit cues of safety through your facial expressions, voice tone, body language, and even subtle physiological signals that others can detect unconsciously. These cues of safety can help trigger other people's nervous systems to move toward regulation as well.

This isn't about being perfect or never experiencing stress. It's about having enough regulation in your own system that you can maintain your grounding even when others around you are struggling. Your regulated presence becomes a resource that others can use to help stabilize their own nervous systems.

Others' regulated states can help regulate you. Just as your calm can influence others, being around regulated people can help your own nervous system settle and find its way back to safety and connection. This is why certain people feel naturally calming to be around, why some relationships leave you feeling more energized and hopeful, and why being part of a supportive community can have such powerful effects on your mental and physical health.

This happens through mirror neurons and unconscious imitation. Your brain contains specialized cells called mirror neurons that fire both when you perform an action and when you observe someone else performing the same action (Rizzolatti & Craighero, 2004). These neurons help you unconsciously mimic the facial expressions, postures, breathing patterns, and even heart rhythms of people you're interacting with.

This mimicry isn't just behavioral - it's physiological. When you unconsciously match someone's relaxed breathing pattern, your own nervous system begins to shift toward the state that pattern represents. When you mirror someone's tense posture, your nervous system responds as if you're experiencing whatever that person is experiencing.

It's why being around anxious people makes you anxious, and calm people help you feel calm. You've probably noticed that anxiety can be contagious - spending time with someone who's worried or stressed often leaves you feeling more worried and stressed yourself, even if their concerns have nothing to do with your life. Similarly, being around someone who's genuinely peaceful and grounded often helps you feel more peaceful and grounded too.

This isn't weakness or lack of boundaries - it's your nervous system doing exactly what it evolved to do. In ancestral environments, matching the emotional and physiological states of your group members helped everyone respond appropriately to threats and opportunities. If someone in your tribe was anxious, there might be good reason for everyone to become more alert. If someone was calm, it might indicate that the environment was safe for everyone to relax.

But here's where it gets interesting in modern contexts: you can learn to work with co-regulation consciously rather than just being at the mercy of whatever nervous system states happen to be around you.

66

You can develop skills for maintaining your own regulation even when others are dysregulated, and you can learn to offer co-regulation support to others when they need it.

Creating Safety for Others

Understanding co-regulation means recognizing that you have the ability to influence other people's nervous system states through your own presence and behavior. This is both a gift and a responsibility - your regulated state can be a powerful resource for others, but it requires developing awareness of how you show up in relationships.

Cues of Safety You Can Offer

Soft eye contact (not staring). Your eyes communicate enormous amounts of information about your internal state and intentions. Soft, appropriate eye contact signals that you're present, engaged, and non-threatening. The key is finding the balance between making enough eye contact to communicate safety and presence without creating intensity that might feel overwhelming or invasive.

Different people have different comfort levels with eye contact based on their cultural background, neurodevelopment, and personal history. The goal isn't to maintain constant eye contact, but to offer the kind of gentle, appropriate visual connection that helps others feel seen and safe.

Genuine, relaxed facial expressions. Your face is constantly communicating information about your nervous system state. When you're genuinely regulated, your facial muscles naturally relax, your expressions become more animated and authentic, and you're more likely to smile in ways that engage your whole face rather than just your mouth.

Forced or fake expressions often backfire because they create incongruence between what you're saying and what your nervous system is actually experiencing. People can detect this mismatch unconsciously, and it often triggers subtle stress responses rather than feelings of safety.

67

Open body posture. Your body language communicates whether you're available for connection or in some form of protective mode. Open postures - uncrossed arms, relaxed shoulders, facing toward the person you're with - signal that you're not defending against threat and that interaction with you is likely to be safe.

This doesn't mean you need to be physically vulnerable or ignore your own safety needs. It means finding ways to communicate openness and availability within whatever boundaries feel appropriate for you and the situation.

Melodic, calm voice tone. The prosodic features of your voice - its rhythm, pitch variation, and tonal qualities - communicate directly to other people's nervous systems. A voice that has natural melody and variation, that isn't rushed or harsh, signals that you're regulated and that interaction with you is likely to be pleasant rather than stressful.

This isn't about speaking in an artificially calm way, but about allowing your natural voice to emerge when you're genuinely in a regulated state. When your nervous system is settled, your voice naturally becomes more melodic and expressive.

Being present rather than rushing. One of the most powerful gifts you can offer another person is your genuine presence - the sense that you're fully here with them rather than thinking about the next thing you need to do. Presence communicates safety because it signals that the current moment is safe enough for you to be fully engaged rather than scanning for threats or planning escapes.

This doesn't mean you need to have endless time for every interaction, but it does mean being fully present for whatever time you do have available.

Protecting Your Own Regulation

Co-regulation works best when you're able to maintain your own nervous system stability while being responsive to others. This requires developing skills for staying grounded in your own regulation even when the people around you are struggling.

When Others Are Dysregulated

Notice your own state first. Before you can offer effective co-regulation support to someone else, you need to know where your own nervous system is. If you're already in sympathetic activation or dorsal shutdown, trying to help someone else regulate often just results in both of you becoming more dysregulated.

This isn't selfish - it's strategic. You can't offer something you don't have. Taking a moment to check in with your own nervous system state helps you determine what kind of support you're actually able to provide.

Take a breath before responding. When someone else is dysregulated, there's often pressure to respond immediately with solutions, reassurance, or action. But taking even one conscious breath before responding can help you stay in your own regulation while choosing a response that's actually helpful rather than reactive.

This pause also gives the other person's nervous system a moment to register your calm presence before you say or do anything, which can sometimes be more helpful than any specific intervention.

Set boundaries if needed. You can't regulate someone who doesn't feel safe with you, and you can't maintain your own regulation if you're consistently overwhelmed by other people's dysregulation. This means sometimes you need to set limits on how much support you can offer or when you can offer it.

Saying something like "I need a moment to think about this" or "I want to help and I need to take care of myself first" allows you to maintain your own regulation while still communicating care for the other person.

You can't regulate someone who doesn't feel safe with you. This is one of the most important principles to understand about co-regulation. If someone's nervous system perceives you as a threat - for any reason, justified or not - your attempts to help them regulate will likely backfire and may actually increase their dysregulation.

This means that sometimes the most helpful thing you can do is step back and allow someone else to provide support, or work on building safety in the relationship before attempting to offer direct regulation support.

Building Regulating Relationships

Understanding co-regulation can help you make more conscious choices about relationships and develop skills for creating the kinds of connections that support everyone's nervous system health.

Look for people who help you feel more like yourself. Pay attention to how you feel during and after spending time with different people. Some relationships will consistently help you feel more grounded, creative, optimistic, or capable, while others might consistently leave you feeling drained, anxious, or disconnected from your own values and preferences.

This information about co-regulation patterns can help you make conscious choices about how to invest your relational energy. It doesn't mean you need to cut off relationships that aren't regulating, but it does mean being strategic about when and how you engage with different people.

Practice being the calm presence you want to encounter. Instead of waiting for other people to provide co-regulation for you, you can develop your own capacity to be a regulating presence for others. This often creates positive feedback loops where your regulation supports others' regulation, which in turn supports your own regulation.

This isn't about being perfect or never struggling. It's about developing the skills to return to regulation relatively quickly and to maintain enough stability to be genuinely helpful to others when they're struggling.

Communicate your needs clearly when possible. Many people assume that others should automatically know how to support their nervous system, but co-regulation actually works better when you can communicate explicitly about what you need. This might mean asking for space when you're overwhelmed, requesting a hug when you need comfort, or letting someone know that you need them to slow down their speech when you're feeling stressed.

Clear communication about nervous system needs helps other people offer more effective support and reduces the guesswork that can create additional stress for everyone involved.

Some relationships may be naturally more dysregulating. Not every relationship will be equally supportive of nervous system regulation, and that's normal. Some people's nervous system patterns, communication styles, or life circumstances may make it difficult for them to offer co-regulation support, regardless of their good intentions.

Understanding this can help you adjust your expectations and develop strategies for managing these relationships without becoming resentful or trying to force changes that aren't realistic.

Neurodiversity Considerations

Co-regulation doesn't look the same for everyone. Individual differences in neurodevelopment, sensory processing, cultural background, and personal history all influence what kinds of interactions feel regulating versus dysregulating.

Co-regulation needs vary greatly between individuals. What feels supportive and regulating for one person might feel overwhelming or uncomfortable for another. Some people regulate best through physical contact, while others need more space. Some people find eye contact essential for feeling connected, while others find it too intense.

Some people regulate better with less eye contact or physical distance. Many neurodivergent individuals, including people with autism, ADHD, or sensory processing differences, may have different co-regulation needs than what's typically expected in social interactions. This doesn't mean they don't benefit from co-regulation - it means they may need different types of support.

71

For example, some people might regulate better through parallel activities (doing something together without direct interaction) rather than face-to-face conversation. Others might prefer text-based communication where they can process and respond at their own pace.

Respect different nervous system needs rather than assuming one approach works for everyone. Effective co-regulation requires paying attention to what actually works for each person rather than applying generic approaches. This might mean asking people directly about their preferences, paying attention to their responses to different types of interaction, or being flexible about how you offer support.

Some people might find it regulating to talk through their feelings, while others might prefer silent companionship. Some might want active problem-solving support, while others need validation and empathy without solutions.

Daily Practice

Developing co-regulation awareness is an ongoing process that you can integrate into your daily interactions and relationships.

Pay attention to how different people affect your nervous system. Start noticing which people consistently help you feel more regulated and which ones tend to activate your stress responses. This isn't about judging people as good or bad, but about gathering information that can help you make conscious choices about relationships.

You might notice that certain people help you feel more creative and optimistic, while others leave you feeling depleted or anxious. Some people might be wonderful in small doses but overwhelming in longer interactions. Others might be supportive during calm times but dysregulating during stressful periods.

Notice without judgment. The goal isn't to categorize people or cut off relationships, but to develop awareness that can inform how you engage with different people. Someone who tends to activate your stress responses might still be an important person in your life - you might just need to interact with them when you're well-resourced or have strategies for maintaining your own regulation during those interactions.

Use this information to make conscious choices. Co-regulation awareness can help you make strategic decisions about relationships and environments. You might choose to spend more time with regulating people when you're going through stressful periods, or you might prepare differently for interactions that you know tend to be activating.

This might also influence choices about work environments, social activities, or living situations. Understanding how different relational contexts affect your nervous system gives you valuable information for creating a life that supports your wellbeing.

The key is using this awareness to support both your own nervous system health and your ability to show up well for the people you care about. When you understand co-regulation, you can be more intentional about offering your regulated presence as a gift to others while also protecting your own capacity to stay grounded and responsive rather than reactive.

Co-regulation represents one of the most powerful tools available for nervous system healing and support. Unlike individual regulation practices that you do alone, co-regulation allows you to access the nervous system resources of others while offering your own resources in return. This creates opportunities for healing and growth that simply aren't available through individual practices alone.

Understanding co-regulation also helps explain why relationships are so central to mental health and wellbeing. It's not just that good relationships make you feel better emotionally - they literally support your nervous system's capacity for regulation, which affects everything from your immune function to your ability to learn and adapt to new challenges.

Chapter 9: Daily Life Applications

Practical Integration Strategies

Now that you understand the basic concepts of polyvagal theory - the three states, neuroception, breathing, movement, sound, and co-regulation - the real question becomes: how do you actually use this information in your everyday life? How do you integrate these insights into the messy, unpredictable, often overwhelming reality of modern living?

The truth is, you don't need to overhaul your entire life or spend hours each day practicing regulation techniques. The most effective approach is usually to start small, focus on consistency rather than perfection, and gradually build nervous system awareness into activities you're already doing.

Think of it this way: your nervous system is constantly active anyway. You're always in some state, always responding to your environment, always co-regulating with the people around you. The goal isn't to add a bunch of new tasks to your already busy life, but to bring more consciousness and choice to processes that are happening whether you pay attention to them or not.

What follows are practical strategies for integrating nervous system awareness into different parts of your day and different areas of your life. These aren't rigid rules but rather starting points for experimentation. Your life circumstances, preferences, and nervous system patterns are unique, so what works for you might look different from what works for others.

The key is to approach this as an ongoing experiment rather than another set of requirements or shoulds. Pay attention to what actually helps you feel more regulated and connected, and don't worry about doing it "right" according to some external standard.

Morning - Setting Your Nervous System Up for Success

How you start your day often influences your nervous system's baseline for the rest of the day. This doesn't mean you need elaborate morning routines or perfect conditions, but small, consistent practices can make a meaningful difference in your overall regulation.

Check in with your state upon waking. Before you reach for your phone, check your email, or start thinking about your to-do list, take just a moment to notice where your nervous system is. Are you waking up feeling rested and alert (ventral vagal), anxious and activated (sympathetic), or groggy and disconnected (dorsal vagal)?

This isn't about judging your state or trying to immediately change it. It's about gathering information that can help you make conscious choices about how to move into your day. If you wake up activated, you might benefit from some gentle movement or breathing before jumping into demanding tasks. If you wake up in shutdown, you might need extra time and gentleness to gradually awaken your system.

Use breathing or gentle movement if needed. Based on your state check-in, you might spend a few minutes with practices that support movement toward regulation. This could be as simple as a few rounds of extended exhale breathing, some gentle stretching in bed, or a short walk around your home.

The goal isn't to force yourself into a particular state, but to support your nervous system in finding its way toward regulation. Sometimes this means calming activation, sometimes it means gently awakening from shutdown, and sometimes it means simply appreciating that you're already regulated.

Eat regularly (blood sugar affects regulation). Your nervous system is exquisitely sensitive to blood sugar fluctuations. When your blood sugar drops, your nervous system often interprets this as a potential threat, which can trigger sympathetic activation or make it harder to maintain regulation throughout the day.

This doesn't mean you need perfect nutrition or elaborate breakfast routines. It means paying attention to how different eating patterns affect your nervous system stability and making choices that support sustained energy rather than dramatic spikes and crashes.

Create predictable morning routines. Your nervous system finds safety in predictability. Having some consistent elements in your morning routine - even if it's just drinking coffee in the same mug or spending five minutes outside - can help signal to your nervous system that you're safe and that the day is starting in a manageable way.

This doesn't mean your routine needs to be rigid or elaborate. It's more about creating some anchoring practices that your nervous system can rely on, especially during stressful periods when everything else might feel uncertain.

Work/School - Navigating Challenges

Your workplace or school environment presents unique challenges for nervous system regulation. You often have limited control over your physical environment, you're required to interact with people whose nervous system states might affect yours, and you may face demanding tasks or deadlines that naturally activate your stress responses.

Before difficult conversations: Breathe and ensure you're in ventral. Challenging conversations - whether it's feedback from a supervisor, a difficult discussion with a colleague, or a presentation to a group - go much better when you start from a regulated state. Taking even one minute to practice calming breathing before these interactions can dramatically improve the outcomes.

When you're in ventral vagal during difficult conversations, you're more likely to listen well, respond thoughtfully rather than reactively, and work toward solutions rather than getting caught in defensive patterns. You're also more likely to help the other person stay regulated through your co-regulation presence.

Email responses: Pause, regulate, then respond. Email can be a particular challenge for nervous system regulation because written communication lacks many of the cues that help us assess safety and threat. It's easy to interpret neutral emails as critical or to respond to challenging emails from activated states.

Developing a practice of pausing before responding to emails - especially ones that trigger immediate emotional reactions - can help you respond from a more regulated place. This might mean taking a breath, checking in with your nervous system state, or even waiting until later in the day to respond if you're feeling particularly activated.

Meetings: Notice your state and others'; use cues of safety. Meetings often involve complex group dynamics that can significantly affect everyone's nervous system states. Paying attention to your own state during meetings can help you stay grounded, while noticing others' states can help you contribute to a more regulated group environment.

You can offer cues of safety during meetings through your presence, voice tone, and body language. Sometimes simply maintaining your own regulation during a tense meeting can help the entire group settle into more productive interaction.

Breaks: 2-minute breathing practices between tasks. Instead of using breaks to check social media or catch up on personal tasks, consider using some of your break time for brief nervous system reset practices. Even two minutes of conscious breathing between demanding tasks can help prevent the accumulation of stress throughout the day.

These mini-practices can be particularly effective during transitions between different types of activities or after particularly challenging interactions.

Evening - Winding Down

The transition from daytime activation to evening rest can be challenging for many nervous systems, especially in our culture where stimulation continues right up until bedtime. Creating supportive evening practices can help your nervous system gradually shift toward the rest and restoration that supports good sleep and next-day regulation.

Transition ritual from work/day stress. Creating some kind of intentional transition between your workday and your evening can help signal to your nervous system that it's time to shift gears. This might be as simple as changing clothes, taking a shower, or spending a few minutes outside.

The specific activity matters less than the intention to create a boundary between the demands of the day and the restoration of the evening. This transition ritual helps your nervous system recognize that it's safe to begin relaxing and that you're moving from productivity mode into rest mode.

Gentle movement or stretching. Evening movement practices are usually most effective when they're calming rather than energizing. Gentle stretching, restorative yoga, or slow walking can help discharge any remaining activation from the day while promoting the kind of calm alertness that transitions well into rest.

The goal isn't to tire yourself out through vigorous exercise, but to help your body settle and release any tension or activation that accumulated during the day.

Calming sounds or music. Using sound strategically in the evening can support your nervous system's transition toward rest. This might mean playing calming music, listening to nature sounds, or even practicing humming or gentle singing.

Many people find that avoiding stimulating sounds - like action movies, intense music, or conflict-heavy news programs - in the evening helps their nervous system settle more effectively.

Connection with family/friends/pets. Positive social connection in the evening can provide valuable co-regulation support while also helping you process the experiences of the day. This might mean sharing meals, having conversations about the day, or simply spending quiet time together.

Connection with pets can be particularly regulating because animals often naturally exist in calm, present states that can help your own nervous system settle.

Conflict Resolution

Understanding nervous system states can dramatically improve how you handle conflicts and disagreements. Most conflicts escalate because one or both people move out of ventral vagal into protective states, which makes productive problem-solving nearly impossible.

Notice if you or the other person has moved out of ventral. The first skill in nervous system-informed conflict resolution is recognizing when someone has moved into sympathetic or dorsal states. Signs might include raised voices, rigid thinking, personal attacks, withdrawal, or statements like "nothing matters" or "what's the point."

Once you can recognize these shifts, you can address the nervous system states before trying to resolve the content of the disagreement.

Pause the content conversation. When nervous systems become dysregulated during conflict, continuing to discuss the original issue usually makes things worse rather than better. Instead of pushing forward with the content, it's often more effective to pause and address the nervous system states first.

This might sound like: "I notice we're both getting pretty activated about this. Can we take a break and come back to it in a few minutes?" or "I want to work this out with you, and I think we'll both think more clearly if we slow down a bit."

Address the nervous system states first. Before returning to the content of the disagreement, take time to help both nervous systems return to regulation. This might involve breathing together, taking a short walk, or simply sitting quietly for a few minutes.

The goal isn't to avoid the conflict or pretend the disagreement doesn't matter. It's to create conditions where both people can access their wisdom, creativity, and capacity for empathy while working through the issue.

Return to problem-solving when both feel calmer. Once both people have returned to more regulated states, you can return to discussing the original issue. You'll often find that solutions emerge more easily, that you can listen to each other more effectively, and that you can work toward outcomes that consider both people's needs.

Parenting Applications

Understanding nervous system regulation can be particularly valuable in parenting because children are still developing their own capacity for regulation and rely heavily on co-regulation with their caregivers.

Regulate yourself first - children co-regulate with your state. This is perhaps the most important principle in nervous system-informed parenting. Your children's nervous systems are constantly reading and responding to your nervous system state. When you're regulated, it's much easier for them to stay regulated. When you're activated or shut down, they're likely to move in similar directions.

This doesn't mean you need to be perfect or never experience stress. It means developing the capacity to return to regulation relatively quickly and to maintain enough stability to be a regulating presence for your children, especially during challenging moments.

Use calm voice and presence during tantrums. Tantrums are often expressions of nervous system overwhelm rather than behavioral problems. Your calm, regulated presence during these moments can help your child's nervous system settle and learn how to manage intense emotions.

This doesn't mean being permissive or ignoring behavior that needs limits. It means staying grounded in your own regulation while providing the co-regulation support your child needs to gradually calm down.

Teach children simple breathing techniques. Children can learn basic breathing practices that help them develop their own capacity for self-regulation. This might be as simple as "belly breathing" (breathing into their belly rather than their chest) or playful practices like blowing bubbles or pretending to smell flowers and blow out candles.

Model healthy responses to stress. Children learn nervous system regulation largely through watching and co-regulating with the adults in their lives. When you model healthy responses to stress - taking deep breaths, asking for help when you need it, taking breaks when you're overwhelmed - you're teaching your children valuable skills for managing their own nervous systems.

Healthcare Settings

Medical and dental appointments often trigger nervous system activation because they involve potential threat (pain, bad news, loss of control) and unfamiliar environments. Understanding your nervous system responses can help you navigate these settings more effectively.

Advocate for your nervous system needs. Many healthcare providers are becoming more aware of how medical environments can trigger stress responses. It's often appropriate to ask for what you need to feel safer - whether that's explanations of procedures, longer appointment times, or modifications to standard protocols.

This might mean requesting that procedures be explained in advance, asking for breaks during long appointments, or requesting that certain lights be dimmed if they feel overstimulating.

Bring a support person if helpful. Having a regulated person with you during medical appointments can provide valuable co-regulation support, especially during stressful procedures or when receiving concerning news.

Support people can also help advocate for your needs if you become overwhelmed or have trouble communicating clearly during medical interactions.

Use breathing techniques during procedures. Many medical and dental procedures become less stressful when you have tools for maintaining nervous system regulation during them. Breathing practices can be particularly helpful because they give you something to focus on while helping your nervous system stay calm.

Communicate with providers about what helps you feel safe. Many healthcare providers want to help patients feel comfortable but may not know what specific individuals need. Communicating clearly about what helps you feel safe and calm can improve your healthcare experiences significantly.

When to Seek Professional Help

While nervous system awareness and regulation practices can be incredibly helpful for many people, some patterns and responses benefit from professional support. Understanding when to seek additional help is an important part of taking care of your nervous system health.

Persistent stuck patterns (always in sympathetic or dorsal). If you find yourself consistently stuck in one nervous system state - always activated and anxious, or always shut down and disconnected - professional support can help you understand what's maintaining these patterns and develop strategies for greater flexibility.

Trauma responses that interfere with daily life. If you're experiencing trauma responses that significantly impact your ability to work, maintain relationships, or engage in activities you value, trauma-informed therapy can provide specialized support for healing nervous system dysregulation related to difficult experiences.

Relationship difficulties related to regulation. Sometimes nervous system patterns create challenges in relationships that benefit from professional guidance. A therapist who understands nervous system functioning can help you and your partners develop better strategies for co-regulation and conflict resolution.

Wanting to explore deeper patterns with support. Even if you're not experiencing crisis-level difficulties, working with a nervous system-informed therapist or coach can help you understand your patterns more deeply and develop more sophisticated regulation skills.

The integration of nervous system awareness into daily life is an ongoing process rather than a destination. The goal isn't to become perfectly regulated or to never experience challenging nervous system states. Instead, it's to develop greater awareness, more conscious choice, and more effective tools for working with your nervous system in ways that support your wellbeing and relationships.

Start small, be patient with yourself, and focus on what actually feels helpful rather than trying to implement every strategy at once. Your nervous system has been taking care of you your entire life - now you have some tools to partner with it more consciously and effectively.

Chapter 10: Integration

What You've Learned

Over the past nine pages, you've gained a practical understanding of how your nervous system works and developed tools for working with it more consciously. You now know about the three basic states your nervous system can inhabit, how it makes decisions about safety and threat through neuroception, and how your breathing, movement, voice, and relationships all influence your nervous system responses.

This isn't just theoretical knowledge - it's practical information that can help you make sense of your own responses and develop more effective strategies for managing stress, building relationships, and moving through your life with greater awareness and choice.

But here's the thing about nervous system work: understanding the concepts is just the beginning. The real value comes from integrating this awareness into your daily life in ways that feel sustainable and helpful rather than overwhelming or perfectionistic.

Your nervous system has been operating for your entire life without your conscious input, and it will continue to function whether you pay attention to it or not. The goal isn't to control or micromanage your nervous system responses, but to develop a partnership with this incredible system that's been working to keep you safe and help you navigate the complexities of being human.

Essential Principles to Carry Forward

Your nervous system responses happen first, stories come second. This might be the most important insight from everything you've learned. Your body makes decisions about safety and threat before your conscious mind knows what's happening. Then your brain creates stories to explain what your body is already experiencing.

Understanding this sequence can help you respond to your own reactions with more curiosity and less judgment. Instead of asking "Why am I being so irrational?" you can ask "What might my nervous system be responding to that I'm not consciously aware of?"

All three states serve important functions. Ventral vagal, sympathetic, and dorsal vagal responses all evolved to help you survive and thrive in different circumstances. The goal isn't to stay in ventral vagal all the time, but to develop the flexibility to move between states as circumstances require and to return to regulation when protective responses are no longer needed.

You can learn to work WITH your nervous system rather than fighting it. Your nervous system isn't broken when it responds in ways that don't make logical sense to your thinking mind. It's doing exactly what it evolved to do based on the information it's receiving and the patterns it's learned from your life experiences.

Working with your nervous system means learning its language, respecting its wisdom, and gently guiding it toward states that serve you better in current circumstances. It's partnership, not domination.

Small, consistent practices create bigger changes than dramatic efforts. Nervous system change happens gradually through repeated experiences of safety and regulation. Brief, regular practices are usually more effective than long, intensive sessions that you can't maintain consistently.

This is about building flexibility and choice, not perfect control. The goal isn't to never experience stress, anxiety, or difficult emotions. It's to develop more conscious choice about how you respond to these experiences and more effective tools for returning to regulation when you're ready.

Daily Practice Suggestions

The most effective way to integrate nervous system awareness is through regular, brief practices that gradually build your capacity for regulation and your awareness of your own patterns.

2-Minute Options

State check-in: "Where am I on the ladder right now?" Throughout your day, simply notice which nervous system state you're experiencing. This isn't about changing anything, just developing awareness of your patterns and what influences them.

You might notice that certain activities, people, or environments consistently affect your nervous system state. This information can help you make more conscious choices about how you structure your time and energy.

Breathing practice when you notice stress. When you notice yourself moving into sympathetic activation or dorsal shutdown, take a minute or two to practice calming breathing. Even a few rounds of extended exhale breathing can help shift your nervous system toward regulation.

Gratitude for something that felt regulating today. Before sleep, briefly acknowledge something that helped you feel more regulated during the day. This might be a conversation that felt connecting, a moment in nature, or simply noticing that you were able to stay calm during a challenging situation.

5-Minute Options

Gentle movement while paying attention to your body. Spend a few minutes moving in whatever way feels good while paying attention to how the movement affects your nervous system state. This might be stretching, walking, dancing, or any other movement that feels supportive.

Intentional connection with someone you care about. Reach out to someone who typically helps you feel more regulated. This might be a text, phone call, or in-person interaction. Pay attention to how the connection affects your nervous system state.

Time in nature or by a window. Spend a few minutes outside or looking out a window, paying attention to natural elements like sky, trees, birds, or weather. Notice how this exposure to nature affects your sense of calm and connection.

10-Minute Options

Combining breathing, movement, and sound. Spend ten minutes integrating multiple regulation practices. You might start with breathing, add some gentle movement, and include humming or listening to calming music.

Journaling about nervous system patterns you noticed. Write briefly about what you noticed regarding your nervous system responses during the day. What triggered movement down the ladder? What helped you feel more regulated? What patterns are you becoming aware of?

Creating a more regulating environment in your space. Spend time adjusting your physical environment to better support nervous system regulation. This might mean organizing, adding plants, adjusting lighting, or arranging furniture in ways that feel more supportive.

Common Pitfalls to Avoid

Making this another way to judge yourself. Nervous system awareness should increase self-compassion, not create new standards for perfection. Your responses make sense given your history and circumstances. The goal is understanding and choice, not judgment.

Expecting instant dramatic changes. Nervous system patterns developed over years or decades don't usually change overnight. Be patient with the process and celebrate small shifts rather than expecting dramatic transformations.

Trying to force yourself into ventral vagal. You can't force regulation any more than you can force yourself to fall asleep. Instead, create conditions that support regulation and allow your nervous system to find its way there naturally.

Ignoring your body's signals in favor of techniques. Your body's wisdom is usually more accurate than any external technique. If a particular practice feels wrong or makes you feel worse, trust that information and try something else.

Using this information to diagnose or fix others. Focus on your own nervous system awareness and regulation. While understanding co-regulation can improve your relationships, trying to diagnose or fix other people's nervous system states usually backfires.

Your Ongoing Journey

Integration of nervous system awareness is a gradual, ongoing process rather than a destination you reach. Your patterns will continue to evolve as you grow and change, and your needs for regulation support may shift based on life circumstances, relationships, and other factors.

This Week

Practice the state check-in daily. Simply begin noticing which nervous system state you're in throughout the day. This basic awareness is the foundation for everything else.

Try one breathing technique. Choose one breathing practice that appeals to you and experiment with using it when you notice stress or activation. Pay attention to how it affects your nervous system state.

Notice one pattern without trying to change it. Pick one situation, relationship, or activity and simply observe how it affects your nervous system. Gather information without pressure to change anything yet.

This Month

Experiment with movement and sound practices. Try different types of movement and sound to see what feels regulating for your nervous system. Build a personalized toolkit of practices that you actually enjoy and find helpful.

Pay attention to your co-regulation patterns. Notice which people and relationships help you feel more regulated and which ones tend to activate stress responses. Use this information to make conscious choices about relationships and social environments.

Begin applying this in one area of life. Choose one area - work, family relationships, or personal self-care - and start consciously applying nervous system awareness. Notice what happens when you bring this consciousness to a specific area of your life.

Ongoing

Develop your personalized toolkit of practices. Over time, you'll discover which specific techniques, activities, and approaches work best for your unique nervous system. Focus on building a sustainable collection of practices rather than trying to use every possible technique.

Share appropriate concepts with family/friends. As you find value in nervous system awareness, you might want to share some concepts with people close to you. Focus on sharing what's been helpful rather than trying to teach or fix others.

Continue learning while staying grounded in what actually helps you. There's always more to learn about nervous system functioning, but stay focused on what actually makes a difference in your daily experience rather than getting lost in theoretical complexity.

Where to Learn More

"Polyvagal Theory in Therapy" by Deb Dana provides practical applications of polyvagal concepts for healing and growth. Dana translates Porges' research into accessible tools for working with nervous system states.

"The Body Keeps the Score" by Bessel van der Kolk explores how trauma affects the nervous system and body, with practical approaches for healing. Van der Kolk integrates polyvagal concepts with other somatic approaches to trauma recovery.

Polyvagal Institute website for scientific updates offers current research and developments in polyvagal theory directly from Stephen Porges and other researchers in the field.

Trauma-informed therapists in your area can provide professional support for working with nervous system patterns, especially if you're dealing with trauma responses or persistent regulation difficulties.

Understanding Yourself Better

This isn't about becoming a different person - it's about understanding the person you already are. Your nervous system has been working to keep you safe your entire life, responding to threats, seeking connection, and adapting to whatever circumstances you've encountered.

Now you have some tools to work with it consciously, compassionately, and effectively. You understand why you respond the way you do in different situations, and you have practical techniques for supporting your nervous system when it needs help returning to regulation.

Your nervous system responses aren't random or broken - they're the result of a sophisticated biological system that's doing its best to help you navigate the complexities of being human. The more you understand this system, the more you can appreciate its wisdom while also guiding it toward responses that serve you well in current circumstances.

Trust your own experience. If something helps you feel more regulated and connected, keep doing it. If it doesn't, try something else. You are the expert on your own nervous system, and you have everything you need to continue learning and growing in partnership with this remarkable system that keeps you alive and helps you thrive.

The journey of nervous system awareness is ongoing, and every small step toward greater understanding and conscious choice makes a difference. Your nervous system has carried you this far - now you can support it in carrying you forward with greater wisdom, compassion, and skill.

Reference

- Breit, S., Kupferberg, A., Rogler, G., & Hasler, G. (2018). Vagus nerve as modulator of the brain-gut axis in psychiatric and inflammatory disorders. *Frontiers in Psychiatry, 9*, 44.

- Brom, D., Stokar, Y., Lawi, C., Nuriel-Porat, V., Ziv, Y., Lerner, K., & Ross, G. (2017). Somatic Experiencing for posttraumatic stress disorder: A randomized controlled outcome study. *Journal of Traumatic Stress, 30*(3), 304–312.

- Brown, R. P., & Gerbarg, P. L. (2005). Sudarshan kriya yogic breathing in the treatment of stress, anxiety, and depression: Part I—neurophysiologic model. *Journal of Alternative & Complementary Medicine, 11*(1), 189–201.

- Brown, R. P., & Gerbarg, P. L. (2012). *The Healing Power of the Breath: Simple Techniques to Reduce Stress and Anxiety, Enhance Concentration, and Balance Your Emotions.* Shambhala Publications.

- Chanda, M. L., & Levitin, D. J. (2013). The neurochemistry of music. *Trends in Cognitive Sciences, 17*(4), 179–193.

- Cohen, S., & Wills, T. A. (1985). Stress, social support, and the buffering hypothesis. *Psychological Bulletin, 98*(2), 310–357.

- Cozolino, L. (2014). *The Neuroscience of Human Relationships: Attachment and the Developing Social Brain.* W. W. Norton & Company.

- Cuddy, A. J., Wilmuth, C. A., Yap, A. J., & Carney, D. R. (2015). Preparatory power posing affects nonverbal presence and job interview performance. *Journal of Applied Psychology, 100*(4), 1286–1295.

- Dana, D. (2018). *The Polyvagal Theory in Therapy: Engaging the Rhythm of Regulation*. W. W. Norton & Company.

- Grossman, P., & Taylor, E. W. (2007). Toward understanding respiratory sinus arrhythmia: Relations to cardiac vagal tone, evolution and biobehavioral functions. *Biological Psychology, 74*(2), 263–285.

- Grossman, P. (2023). Fundamental challenges and likely refutations of the five basic premises of the polyvagal theory. *Biological Psychology, 176*, 108467.

- Holt-Lunstad, J., Smith, T. B., & Layton, J. B. (2010). Social relationships and mortality risk: A meta-analytic review. *PLOS Medicine, 7*(7), e1000316.

- Jerath, R., Edry, J. W., Barnes, V. A., & Jerath, V. (2006). Physiology of long pranayamic breathing: Neural respiratory elements may provide a mechanism that explains how slow deep breathing shifts the autonomic nervous system. *Medical Hypotheses, 67*(3), 566–571.

- Kang, J., Scholp, A., & Jiang, J. J. (2018). A review of the physiological effects and mechanisms of singing. *Journal of Voice, 32*(4), 390–395.

- Kaplan, R., & Kaplan, S. (1989). *The Experience of Nature: A Psychological Perspective*. Cambridge University Press.

- Li, Q. (2010). Effect of forest bathing trips on human immune function. *Environmental Health and Preventive Medicine, 15*(1), 9–17.

- Nestor, J. (2020). *Breath: The New Science of a Lost Art*. Riverhead Books.

- Pascoe, M. C., Thompson, D. R., & Ski, C. F. (2017). Yoga, mindfulness-based stress reduction and stress-related physiological measures: A meta-analysis. *Psychoneuroendocrinology, 86*, 152–168.

- Porges, S. W. (2004). Neuroception: A subconscious system for detecting threats and safety. *Zero to Three, 24*(5), 19–24.

- Porges, S. W. (2011). *The Polyvagal Theory: Neurophysiological Foundations of Emotions, Attachment, Communication, and Self-regulation.* W. W. Norton & Company.

- Rizzolatti, G., & Craighero, L. (2004). The mirror-neuron system. *Annual Review of Neuroscience, 27,* 169–192.

- Schore, A. N. (2001). Effects of a secure attachment relationship on right brain development, affect regulation, and infant mental health. *Infant Mental Health Journal, 22*(1–2), 7–66.

- Schore, A. N. (2003). *Affect Regulation and the Repair of the Self.* W. W. Norton & Company.

- Thayer, J. F., & Lane, R. D. (2009). Claude Bernard and the heart–brain connection: Further elaboration of a model of neurovisceral integration. *Neuroscience & Biobehavioral Reviews, 33*(2), 81–88.

- Thayer, J. F., Åhs, F., Fredrikson, M., Sollers III, J. J., & Wager, T. D. (2012). A meta-analysis of heart rate variability and neuroimaging studies: Implications for heart rate variability as a marker of stress and health. *Neuroscience & Biobehavioral Reviews, 36*(2), 747–756.

- van der Kolk, B. A. (2014). *The Body Keeps the Score: Brain, Mind, and Body in the Healing of Trauma.* Viking.

- Zaccaro, A., Piarulli, A., Laurino, M., Garbella, E., Menicucci, D., Neri, B., & Gemignani, A. (2018). How breath-control can change your life: A systematic review on psycho-physiological correlates of slow breathing. *Frontiers in Human Neuroscience, 12,* 353.

www.ingramcontent.com/pod-product-compliance
Lightning Source LLC
Chambersburg PA
CBHW050547280326
41933CB00011B/1755